HOW TO OVERCOME CONSTIPATION, A TOXIC COLON AND DIARRHOEA ONCE AND FOR ALL

WITH NATURAL FOOD INGREDIENTS AND WITHOUT THE USE OF LAXATIVES

(AND WHY DIARRHOEA MIGHT BE A FORM OF CONSTIPATION)

by Peter Jackson

Published by
The Healthy Bowels Publishing Company
Marston Green
Birmingham
B33 0NW
Tel: +44 (0) 121 779 6619
Fax: +44 (0) 121 779 3110

Printed and Bound in Great Britain

ISBN 978-0-9564011-0-6

CONTENTS

CONTENTS

CONTENTS

CHAPTER 1
Introduction

This book can change your life dramatically for the better.

There are two reasons why I can make this statement so confidently.

Firstly, there is a growing opinion in Naturopathic circles that your health begins in your colon. In other words, if you can keep your bowels clean and healthy then you are more likely to be able to keep disease in other parts of the body at bay.

Put another way – many believe that most diseases that develop do so as the result of a 'dirty' colon. The assumption is therefore that a 'clean' colon will go a long way to preventing disease developing in other parts of the body.

Secondly, the great thing about the diet I recommend in this book is that it is not only good for your bowels – it's also good for the overall health of your body.

You see, the diet that is going to cleanse your digestive system will also help cleanse your tubes in other parts of your body – like your arteries.

And the adjustments I am going to be recommending are simple to do.

We are not talking about a whole lot of new foods in your diet. All I am recommending is that you change the balance.

This does not mean hardship and it does not mean hunger.

It means consuming a wider range of natural live foods which you will enjoy and getting rid of a lot of 'dead' harmful foods.

Your new cleansing diet will mean you will feel better and have more energy. You will have a digestive system that flows freely – without straining or unnatural urgency.

My own personal interest in bowel health started nearly 20 years ago when I suffered from a 'three year spell' of Irritable Bowel Syndrome.

My experience at that time taught me that, to a great extent, your health is in your hands and it is your responsibility to look after yourself because no-one else is going to do that for you.

And that means understanding the power of food and how it can help keep your body healthy.

'You are what you eat' may be an old saying but, like most sayings, it has a major element of truth in it.

My experience with my own bowel problem also taught me that your overall health revolves around your digestive system.

I was lucky – I had been involved in the complementary health trade for some years by that time and I had access to some very helpful and knowledgeable naturopaths.

I soon learned that certain foods and natural food ingredients could have a direct effect on my bowel health.

After some experimentation, I was able to develop a combination of natural food ingredients and foods that could help me to overcome my Irritable Bowel Syndrome.

I am happy to say that these same ingredients have kept me symptom free for the last ten years and this has led me to establish my own company to offer those natural nutrients that had helped me, to a much wider audience.

Over the last ten years, I have spoken to, and worked with, many hundreds of people suffering from every type of bowel ailment you can think of.

There is one bowel disease however that rides above all in terms of commonality – one ailment that most of us in the West seem to suffer from in one way or another – that of debilitating constipation.

If this is a problem that you are suffering from – and it is probably fairly safe to assume so or otherwise you would not be reading this – then help is at hand.

Because of my own experiences and the business I have run over the last ten years, I have taken a particular interest in those foods and natural nutrients that can overcome your constipation once and for all – in a natural way – without any side-effects.

The aim of this book is to pass on my findings to you. I hope you enjoy it.

But before starting, I thought I might list below some statements I picked up whilst doing my research. As you might expect, these statements relate to bowel health or should I say bowel disease.

- *'Poor digestion overburdens the metabolism of every cell and leads to changes in the cell's efficiency, the resilience of the connective tissue and the skin. It puts excessive strain on the primary organs of metabolism such as the liver, kidneys and intestines. Our entire body can become overloaded with harmful substances.'*

- *'There are two types of constipation. One type is present when the faeces that pass from the body are overly packed together. Another type of constipation is present when old, hardened faeces stick to the walls of the colon and do not pass out with regular bowel movements. Both types of constipation are so common among the members of modern society today that scarcely anybody recognises them as being unnatural.'*

- *'It is estimated that poor digestion and elimination is to blame for a host of modern ailments, yet most of these are preventable.'*

- *'Most middle aged people have between three and fifteen pounds of undigested faecal matter stuck in their colon. Waste matter which gets stuck in the colon is highly toxic, and can suppress the immune system, potentially causing gas, bloating and constipation, dramatically reducing the assimilation of nutrients and slowing metabolism.'*

- *'Chronic diseases build up over a long period of time. About 80 percent of the patients who go to the doctors have chronic diseases. The American Cancer Society says it takes twenty years to develop cancer. What are people developing in their body today? Never underestimate the value of a clean colon.'*

All of us, as we get older, will have some sort of build up in our tubes whether it is in our arteries or digestive tract. The secret to good health is to keep these tubes from getting so blocked up that they literally 'choke' your body to death.

Constipation is a western problem. And now, so are IBS, Diverticulitis, laxative addiction, anal fissures, haemorrhoids, sluggishness, fatigue, bloating and so on. Is this just a coincidence?

Happy reading.

CHAPTER 2

Why the natural colic gastric reflex of our ancestors has been lost

Not a question you get asked every day, but how often do you go?

It appears that the average transit time we have in the UK and in Europe in general, from the time food goes into your mouth to the time waste matter is expelled at the other end is far too long.

It should be no more than 24 hours at most but, for many, it can be 60 hours or even in some cases much, much, much longer.

Our rural African counterparts can go up to 3 times per day, almost after each meal.

That's in keeping with the gastro-colic reflex that has evolved over thousands and thousands of years.

That means that after each meal, when your stomach is full, a message is sent down to your bowels to evacuate its contents to make room for more on its way down.

It's a natural process but one which few of us in the UK, it seems, experience very much at all.

How often should you go? Most doctors would advocate at least one good bowel movement a day. Natural Practitioners would probably say 2-3 times per day.

The important thing is that you should be able to pass well formed, soft stools that are not difficult to pass on a fairly regular basis.

The first sign for most people that their digestive system is clogged is when constipation and the passing of motions becomes a problem. Diarrhoea might also be a problem that is related to a clogged system as well.

The typical reaction in situations like this is for people to focus only on their bowels to overcome the problem. This might mean adding more bran fibre to the diet (quite often the second last thing you should do) or going to the chemist to get some laxatives (often the last thing you should do). In the case of diarrhoea, the option might also be to go for a quick fix, rather than looking at what is causing the symptoms in the first place.

I will devote more time to diarrhoea later as quite often it can be the result of a clogged system that is not functioning properly. In other words, many cases of diarrhoea – if more serious problems have been ruled out by your doctor - might be a form of constipation.

Why constipation and a toxic colon are not just a bowel problem, they could be caused by a weakened digestive system

For most people who suffer from a constipated system, the problem has probably started higher up in the digestive tract where food has not been broken down properly and therefore not digested efficiently, thus making it more difficult for the colon to handle and eliminate.

So, constipation is not just about your bowels and it's not just about fibre either. There's a whole list of things that have probably caused your system to be clogged and bloated.

If you want to overcome constipation naturally then the starting point has to be, understand the causes in the first place. Once you know these, you can then take the necessary action required to overcome the problem once and for all without having to resort to the 'quick and temporary' fix of a laxative.

This is the aim of this book – to help all of you who are suffering from constipation and intermittent diarrhoea to overcome these distressing conditions once and for all.

The word constipate in Latin, constipare, means press together. A constipated bowel is one where the faeces are packed solidly together.

So, the first thing is to look at what causes faeces being packed tightly together.

There is a growing body of opinion in naturopathic circles which believes that in the UK, and the West in general, our diets have not only become deprived of natural, healthy fibre, it has also become too mucus forming and a far cry from the diet of our ancestors.

So, quite a large part of this book will be devoted to looking at how an overproduction of mucus in our digestive system could be one of the causes of a clogged up, toxic colon.

I will also be talking about fibre of course, as you can't talk about bowels without talking about fibre.

But, did you know that one of the most common fibres consumed could in fact be one of the major contributors to mucus in your system and therefore one of the potential causes of constipation?

I will be looking at this in more detail as well.

Diets like most things in life, are all about balance. Most of us in the UK have the pendulum swinging too much in the favour of a mucus diet instead of one that is more cleansing, and mucus free. With some adjustments to your diet and help from some natural ingredients, where appropriate, we can get your bowels working again without having to resort to laxatives or enemas. By changing the emphasis in your diet, we can get it to have more of a natural 'cleansing' effect in your system rather than a 'clogging' effect.

Laxatives can make a constipated situation worse

If you do take laxatives then, beware, they can only make a constipated situation worse. Any type of stimulant, natural or otherwise, works by artificially kick-starting the bowel into an unnatural peristalsis action (the muscular contractions of the large bowel which propel waste matter through to expulsion). Over time, your system can come to rely on these stimulants. Also, laxatives do nothing whatsoever to clean and clear your bowels they just encourage the bowels to evacuate what is in the system at any one time. They do nothing to break down the hardened waste matter that might have accumulated.

Levels of constipation vary from individual to individual. You can get mild constipation such as when you go on holiday and a change of diet throws your digestive rhythm out. You can then go right to the other end of the scale when a build up of toxic waste has clogged up the whole digestive system over many years. This is what I often refer to as 'middle aged constipation.' This is a lot tougher to deal with as impacted waste can be 'crusty' and hard and firmly attached to the digestive tract. It can make it difficult to absorb nutrients from your food and for your colon to do its job and expel waste.

In situations like this, you need to tackle the problem from every angle.

Why Jamie Oliver was right about rural Africans

At the beginning of this book, I referred to rural Africans who are known to defecate up to three times per day - far more than we do in the UK. As they have virtually no bowel disease, it's worth taking a look at their diets in more detail. Of course, their lifestyle could be said to be far less stressful than ours and so this also has to be taken into consideration, but for the sake of this book we are going to focus on food.

Jamie Oliver managed to demonstrate on television quite graphically how their bowel habits differ to ours.

In the television studio, he had a large vat of brown stuff (virtual poo) which represented what the average rural African passed in one year. By its side, in a vat that was around one third of the size, was what the average person in the UK passed. This visual comparison was quite staggering and a wake-up call to many watching.

The main issue here is that if, as it is suggested, we eat more calories than our African counter parts, and they are passing 3 to 4 times more waste than us, what happens to all that other waste that we should be passing? Where is it going?

This is the question that more and more naturopaths ask and perhaps it is one that you should as well.

Many experts believe impacted waste material in the bowel can harden and thicken over the years restricting the colon passage.

So, why are we not passing as much waste matter as rural Africans, even though our calories are much higher?

These are the questions I want to address.

But it's not only adults who are suffering. It's younger people as well.

What surprises me is the number of young people who seem to get constipation these days. I suppose it shouldn't surprise me when you look at the amount of fast food many of them eat. It contains little or no fibre and is comprised of what I describe as 'clogging' foods like white bread and dairy. Also, I notice that children eat a far less varied diet today than that of my parents when they were young.

Young girls can be particularly vulnerable to constipation when they go on low fat, low calorie diets.

The size of the laxative market demonstrates the massive problem constipation has become, and it seems to be getting worse.

Don't become one of the statistics

I read one survey recently which suggested that bowel health was low on most peoples' priority list. So, if you are one of these who is not convinced that going to the loo regularly is that important, take a look at some of these statistics:

- 12% of deaths in the UK are linked to the digestive tract.
- 1 in 8 of all admissions to general hospitals in the UK are associated with digestive diseases and conditions.
- 1 in 4 main operations within general hospitals are performed on the digestive tract.
- 5% of British adults suffer from long-standing illness of the digestive tract.
- Over a third of the population regularly suffers from digestive illnesses such as Irritable Bowel Syndrome, constipation, diarrhoea, stomach-aches, nausea and sickness.
- GPs prescribe over £800 million worth of drugs for the gastrointestinal system every year in England, Northern Ireland and Scotland.

What to look out for

- Bowel cancer is the 3rd most diagnosed cancer and 2nd commonest cause of cancer death in the UK.
- Cancers of the digestive tract are the largest cancer killer, accounting for 23% of all UK cancer mortalities.
- Coeliac disease is very common in the west, but virtually unknown elsewhere in the world. In Britain there is high incidence, with 1 in 1000 people affected.
- Over 3 million people in the UK suffer from constipation every month.
- An estimated 200 million people around the world, on any given day, suffer from diarrhoea.
- Over half of over-70's in the UK have diverticula, a disease of the large intestine.

- About one in ten people in Britain have gallstones, especially women, overweight people, and those who are middle aged or over.

- Faecal incontinence (soiling) may affect 1 in 20 people.

- 2 million people are hit every year by food poisoning.

- Irritable Bowel Syndrome is very common, affecting a third of our population at one time or another. About 1 in 10 people suffer symptoms bad enough to go to a doctor.

- About half the population has haemorrhoids by the age of 50.

- Ulcers are common in Britain. About 1 in 10 men and 1 in 5 women suffer from an ulcer at some time in their lives. In most people they heal up with treatment.

- Stomach cancer is the 5th most common cancer for men in the UK and the 6th for women

- Ulcerative Colitis & Crohn's disease affects 150,000 people in the UK, with 8,500 new cases being diagnosed every year.

The purpose of this book is to help you to avoid being one of these statistics. For this to happen, your stools should be soft and bulky and easy to pass.

In other words: Big stools, small hospitals!

I mentioned earlier that constipation, in most cases, does not start in the colon. It probably starts earlier on in the digestive process.

For this reason, in chapter three, I want to take a closer look at higher up the digestive system.

But, before doing that, let's take a little diversion to look at why it is not only food that is causing our clogged up bowels.

CHAPTER 3

Holding on – why we in the UK like to hold on to our waste matter

Why your upbringing can be encouraging you to be constipated

Do you remember how things were when you were a child at school? There were certain times when you were supposed to go to the loo.

At my country primary school, even when we were very young, we were programmed to go to the loo at specific times.

I recall many 'accidents' at school because children were restricted to going at certain times.

This is not how the digestive system should be programmed. You should never fight the urge to go. When you feel like going, you should go.

Instead of going three times per day, as many natural practitioners believe you should, most of us are programmed to go only once per day - usually first thing in the morning -when you are often rushing to get out to work after a rushed breakfast.

This is totally at odds with the natural colic reflex I mentioned in Chapter two where the digestive system was programmed, many years ago, to empty its bowels after every meal to make room for waste food on its way down.

So, gradually over the last few generations, for most of us, the natural stomach-colic reflex has been snuffed out.

My generation was brought up not talking about going to the loo. It was a taboo subject.

I remember the headmaster at my primary school getting really embarrassed when he had to talk about defecation. Because it was never discussed, going to the loo was never encouraged. Holding on to waste matter was not considered a problem.

In fact it appears there are many people of my generation who 'hold on' to their waste matter not only for the way we were brought up but in many cases for psychological reasons. I'm not going into that in this book, but 'suppression' is endemic in many of my generation.

Because of this ignorant and rather Victorian attitude, people who were born in the 1950's didn't think twice about suppressing evacuation if they were busy or it was inconvenient – particularly if they were away from home.

Women in particular appear to be guilty of this. I have heard of cases where women have hardly gone to the loo for two weeks whilst away on holiday because they didn't like going to the loo in a strange place or when they were sharing with friends.

So we must always fight this urge to hold on when things are not convenient. It is bad enough that there are so many common foods that we eat that are literally 'choking' our systems to death. Making things worse by suppressing the urge to go is the last thing we should be doing.

Does it always have to be first thing in the morning?

I find that many people are fixated about having to go to the loo before they leave the house for work or at least some time in the morning. If things are not moving through smoothly then frustration can set in and lead to straining which if, continued over a period of time, can lead to haemeorrhoids and diverticular disease.

Of course, if you can go nice and easily first thing, that's great. If you can't then it might be worth considering different times of the day to sit on the loo.

Try to find a time when you are not going to be rushed. Evenings, such as after your evening meal is worth a try if this is a quiet time for you. You can sit there with a good magazine! Then, over a period of time, you might be able to re-kindle your natural rhythm.

Bet you've never thought of squatting

One thing we could probably learn from our ancestors is that they squatted when evacuating their bowels. By squatting, I mean that their knees were higher than their hips. This was obviously natural for them as they would just 'squat' whenever the call to nature came.

Squatting is a more effective position to adopt to evacuate your bowels effectively.

Now before I hear you say that you can't stand on the toilet seat at your age, there are simple ways you can adopt a squatting position.

One is to put two or three thick books or a small kitchen stool in front of the loo so that when you sit down, you can raise your knees above your hips. It may feel a bit strange to begin with, but stay with it and you will find that it really helps for a more thorough evacuation of the bowels.

As I emphasise throughout this book, your bowels do not work in isolation. They are the final part of your digestive system and how they function may often be reliant on how well you cope with digesting your food further up.

So, before proceeding to look at your diet in more detail, I would like to take a cursory look around your digestive system.

CHAPTER 4

A Quick Look Around Your Digestive System

To get to the bottom of this constipation problem, so to speak, and to find how things might go wrong, let's take a look at the complete digestive process which starts in your mouth when you start chewing your food.

The perfect digestive system

Let's assume that your digestive system, from the moment you put food into your mouth, to the point of exit from your rectum runs pretty smoothly. You don't get indigestion, excess acid, bad breath, bloating, excess wind or foul smelling stools. Instead you have good, soft bowel movements two to three times a day.

If your digestive system performed like that then your diet must have been pretty perfect for the previous 20 years or so!

This means that the majority of your diet has been made up primarily of fresh fruit and vegetables. Fish would be eaten perhaps three to four times per week.

You would only be eating red meat, at most, once per month and wheat and dairy would make up no more than 5% of your diet.

Off the menu totally would have been pastries, processed meats and cakes.

You would have been chewing your food many times before swallowing (it would be totally liquid). Whilst you have been chewing so efficiently, the food has mixed thoroughly with enzymes that help break down carbohydrates for absorption.

You would have then swallowed this liquid which, once in your stomach, would release lots of acid and other enzymes that help break down protein in your food.

As your food is liquid anyway (because you have chewed it so well) this process is performed with no strain or indigestion.

This liquid is then passed through the small intestine where, because it has been broken down so well in the stomach, is ready to be absorbed through the thousands of millions of microvillus present in the small intestine which are responsible for the absorption of very tiny nutrients. Eighty percent of nutrient absorption takes place in the small intestine.

This whole process is aided by cells on the microvillus that secrete mucus to help lubricate the digestive tract making it easier for food not wanted for digestion to slip through to the colon. Their job is made so much easier as you have chewed your food so well and any protein content has been totally liquidised in the stomach.

The intestine and large bowel wall are pink and healthy with no waste build up on the sides, making passage of liquid food and waste matter unrestricted.

The 'sludge' that then makes its way into the large bowel or colon is fairly slimy but not at all 'sticky' which makes it easy for the bowels to handle.

The main role of the colon is to re-absorb water from the sludge and make waste material, which is being formed into moist stools, ready for elimination. Because the stools are moist and free from 'stodgy' mucus there is no effort or straining on elimination.

Does that apply to you?

My guess is that there are very few of us who have digestive systems like that. The fact is that if you lived in rural Africa and you lived like a native and ate like them, you would have a far better chance of having a perfect digestive system than those of us living in Europe or the USA.

This brief look at the digestive system is to demonstrate how your digestive system is connected and in very basic terms how it should function.

Quite often people who have been constipated for many years not only end up with bowel diseases such as diverticular disease and haemorrhoids but the 'backing up' of waste matter can cause pressure on the digestive system further up and so everything can get clogged including other organs like the gall bladder and the lymphatic system.

Alternatively, you may start off with problems of indigestion first and then find some time later that you are not evacuating your bowels as often as you used to.

A hiatus hernia is not uncommon in people who have been constipated for many years although rarely are the two connected.

So, if you digest your food well then this gives things further on in the process a better chance of working more smoothly.

I wanted to look at your whole digestive system first to emphasise the fact that your bowels don't work in isolation. If we can take a more panoramic view of things then, hopefully, this will give you a better chance of success rather than trying to find a quick fix with an antacid for heartburn, a laxative for constipation or something to slow down diarrhoea.

If the digestive system is clear and slippery then things can pass through unhindered. Unfortunately there are many aspects of our diets and our lifestyle that prevent this from happening.

Why your diet could be choking your digestive system to 'death'

Instead, it is not unusual for European people, particularly when we get to middle age, to have a digestive system that is 'sticky' and clogged up - anything but slippery and clear.

A clogged up system does not only mean constipation. It can also mean diarrhoea where the digestive tubes becomes so clogged with layers of rubbish that waste matter just shoots through. This means that the digestive tract is unable to do its work of absorbing nutrients efficiently in the small intestine and reabsorbing liquid from waste matter in the large intestine.

We take good digestion for granted, but many people suffer routinely from poor digestion. Most of us recognise at least some of the symptoms – wind, bloating, constipation, diarrhoea and stomach pains. But there are other less obvious signs. These can include lowered immunity, allergic reactions, skin problems, slow healing of wounds, lack of energy and chronic fatigue and candidiasis.

I have only taken a cursory look at the digestive system, but I want you to link how you chew and process your food to what eventually happens in your bowels. The better you understand this, the better you will be able to sort out your constipation once and for all.

I'm now going to talk quite a bit about digestive enzymes because they are SO important for the whole digestive process.

Enzymes and how your digestion works

Digestion breaks food down so it can be absorbed into the body. This process begins even before we put food in our mouth. Just the sight and smell of food makes your mouth 'water' and triggers saliva production. Once you begin chewing, saliva helps lubricate the food, and enzymes in the saliva start the process of digesting carbohydrates (or starch).

Now you swallow the food and it reaches your stomach. Here the gastric juices are secreted. These juices contain acids and protein-digesting enzymes. Animal protein is hard work for these enzymes to break down, so a steak or slice of cheese may stay in your stomach for several hours before moving down to the small intestine.

Here, enzymes that digest carbohydrates and fats are released into the small intestine. The nutrients extracted from the food we have eaten include vitamins, minerals, amino acids, sugars and fatty acids – all essential to health. These are then absorbed into the body as the food travels down the long length of your small intestine. By the time food reaches the colon, most of what your body needs has already been absorbed. Anything left is waste, to be excreted.

Many of us might not be producing important enzymes that we need to digest different types of food. If you have a dairy intolerance then you may not be producing the lactase enzyme which is responsible for breaking down lactose in milk. But the enzymes we need to digest our food properly are not only about what our own bodies secrete themselves, it is also about what enzymes are present in food - or should I say are not present.

For this reason you might find it interesting to learn a little bit about the history of our food and their enzyme activity. There's a bit of technical stuff here, but it is worth taking note of.

Why your food contains less enzymes.

As well as being produced by the body, digestive enzymes are found in raw food. In fact, all raw food naturally contains the proper types and proportions of enzymes needed to digest itself. But when you cool or store food for any length of time, the enzymes are destroyed or degraded, so that your body has the task of producing the enzymes that it needs. Over time, this may tax our digestive processes too heavily, and food may not be broken down efficiently. If nutrients are poorly absorbed we can end up with digestive discomfort, food allergies and even malnutrition.

Enzymes are like tiny robots working in an assembly line; they help break down or build up body chemicals, and each has a very specific job. Each enzyme digests a particular type of food, breaking it down so it can be easily absorbed through the digestive walls.

Proteins, for example are broken down by proteases and peptidase. Carbohydrates, which include sugars and starches, are tackled by enzymes with names like amylase, invertase, malt diastase and glucoamylase. Fats are split down by lipase. To digest plant fibres found in grains, fruit and vegetables the body needs cellulose, which it can't make for itself. If milk and milk products give you digestive discomfort, as I have mentioned before, you may be suffering from a lack of lactase, the enzyme that breaks down milk sugar or lactose.

A lack of digestive enzymes can lead to allergy hazards

If enzymes are lacking our nutritional intake will, of course, suffer. Food remaining undigested will putrefy, encouraging the wrong kind of bacteria and lead to wind, bloating, inflammation and stomach pains. Worse, these conditions can create a 'leaky gut' – literally holes in the digestive lining that allow incompletely digested food into the bloodstream. More details of this are given in Chapter 6.

Therefore, if you have been constipated for a long while, take a look first at your digestive system higher up. If you suffer from indigestion, stomach acid and bloating you may be having difficulty in handling certain types of foods. Food that enters your small intestine not properly broken down can be treated as a 'foreign invader,' causing your body to produce mucus secretions. This reaction can prove to be the starting point in the clogging of your digestive system and ultimately your constipation. It can be one of the key reasons why your system can get more constipated.

Food enzymes are so important, therefore, to help prevent this clogging process from getting going in the first place. However, we are unable to rely on our foods to supply them in the way that they did many years ago.

As previously mentioned, due to the way that we process and produce our fresh foods these days, our vegetables are not so 'alive' with enzymes as they used to be. Over time, this can put a strain on our own systems to produce more enzymes than they would normally expect.

It is for this reason, I would recommend that those people who are plagued with constipation would benefit by taking a natural digestive enzyme supplement. I talk more about this in Chapter 10.

But of course it's not only important that your digestive system is working properly, it is also important to put the right food into it in the first place.

So, the next stage is to look at our diets and find out just what pressurises our systems to grind to a halt in the first place, leaving our bodies open to disease and why one type of fibre might, in fact, be a cause of constipation.

CHAPTER 5

Why one fibre in particular may be one of the causes of your constipation

I would imagine that you, like everyone else on this planet, have heard that you need to eat more fibre if you have constipation and no-one can argue with that.

There are many ways to get your extra fibre. Getting them from natural fresh vegetables, beans, pulses, whole grains and fruit is of course the best way because you get fibre in its natural state with other nutrients. Of course, for those people who have severe constipation which may have developed over many years, simply adding extra fruit and veg to the diet does not always do the trick.

'I have changed my diet and increased my fibre but I still don't go properly!'

I have heard from many, many people who are frustrated by the fact that they have changed their diets to take in lots of extra fibre but find they still have no improvement in their bowel habits. In fact many increase wheat bran when wheat may have been one of the contributors to constipation in the first place.

So, for cases like this, a more radical change to the diet may be needed.

Many will go for a quick fix if a new diet doesn't yield good results quickly. The obvious quick fix is the artificial laxative from the chemist. This, as I have said before, is not an option if you really want to find a solution that is going to be long-lasting as it will only make things worse.

Even so-called natural laxatives that contain senna are really not much better and should not be taken long-term. Many laxative products on the market try to give a 'natural feel' to the product by disguising the fact that they contain a stimulating herb like senna. Make sure you check the ingredient list if unsure.

Often the second choice of 'quick fix' is to add lots of bran fibre. This is fine for a short term effect but in the long term the bran fibre, because of its abrasive nature, might prove to be too harsh for some. Also it doesn't 'cleanse' the system like some other forms of fibre. But the other problem with bran fibre is that it can contain gluten, a protein that might be one of the causes of your digestive system getting 'bunged up.'

Why you might be 'overdosing' on gluten.

Bran fibre comes from wheat and since the 1970's there has been a major increase in the consumption of wheat products as many people perceive that this is a good way of getting in extra fibre.

The problem is that wheat, because of the gluten it contains, may actually be contributing to the clogging of your digestive systems and your constipation.

These days, wheat is present in so much of our food that we are literally 'overdosing' on gluten, the protein found in wheat.

I am going to go into more detail on this in the next chapter but, for the moment, let's take a quick look at two main types of fibre.

Why soluble fibre is emerging as the fibre in the 21st century

Apparently there are five different types of fibre, but you will find there are two you will hear about most, they are soluble and insoluble fibre.

In short, bran fibre like wheat bran is classified as insoluble fibre. It is known as 'roughage.' It is not so water retentive but can stimulate bowels by a natural process of 'scratching' the bowel wall as it moves through, therefore stimulating a peristalsis movement.

Whereas this process is perfectly natural, you can imagine that this 'scratching' effect could make a sensitive situation worse.

Soluble fibre by contrast has more absorbent qualities and tends to be more water retentive and therefore more viscous. This viscous quality makes it more 'gentle' on the digestive system and, in most cases, it is better for people with sensitive bowels than insoluble fibre. A typical example of soluble fibre is oats.

Soluble fibre in general is the best sort of fibre because it has a more 'cleansing' effect than insoluble fibre. Soluble fibre is also good for helping keep blood sugar stable and cholesterol levels in check – one of the reasons why, in the USA, they are advocating that everyone eat lots more soluble fibre.

Over the last 100 years our demands for, and interest in, fibre have gone through some changes. Here is a very brief summary of what has been going on.

A brief history of fibre in the 20th Century!!

Our grandparents and their parents enjoyed far higher levels of fibre in their diet because they ate a lot more fresh food with higher levels of naturally occurring fibre. The advantage of getting fibre in this way is that high fibre foods like whole grains contain not only lots of fibre but also other beneficial nutrients and antioxidants.

The bread they consumed would have been from whole wheat. However, overall, wheat played a much smaller role in their diets than it does in ours today. Also, the nature of our wheat has changed. The wheat we consume today is much harder for our digestive systems to cope with.

In the 1930's and 1940's, white bread became fashionable and fibre almost became a forgotten word. White bread was even considered by many to be better for you than whole wheat.

Despite this lapse, people were still eating lots more fresh food than today and this provided, in most cases, sufficient levels of fibre.

It wasn't until the 1970's that we started to think about fibre supplements. It was then that a Dr Birkett from the UK started to study the diet of rural Africans who had virtually no bowel disease, compared to Western Europe where the disease was increasing.

To cut a long story short, Dr Birkett discovered the main difference between the two diets was the level of fibre. Needless to say, the levels of fibre in the black African diet were far higher than the western diet. Their fibre came mainly from whole grains which also had the benefits of extra, naturally occurring nutrients. It didn't come just from whole wheat or wheat bran.

After this study and his book were published, people started to eat more fibre and went for the second 'quick fix'. This meant buying big bags of wheat bran fibre from the health shop to add to their cereals even though this was missing the point of the research that most of the fibre came from natural foods, not extracted wheat bran.

Nevertheless, this new development started people thinking that they could overcome their constipation by a quick fix of adding extra wheat bran – little knowing that this could in fact be making their constipation worse in the long run.

The wheat bran trend continued into the 1980's when the demand for fibre exploded with the publication of The F Plan Diet. It was at this time that fibre supplements were launched as an aid for weight loss. Once again, these supplements tended to be based on wheat and insoluble fibre.

Then the 90's came with more written about low fat and low calorie diets and fibre once again took a back seat.

The emphasis is now on soluble fibre

Since 2000, fibre has made a big comeback in the USA and this has started to filter through over here in the UK. This time the news is not so much about insoluble fibre, it's all to do with soluble fibre.

In the USA, the general recommendation is that everyone should consume 35-55g of fibre per day and the emphasis is definitely on soluble fibre. It is stated that most people consume less than half of this. (Not surprising when you look at the average fast food diet in the USA.)

The American authorities are trying to get people to consume more soluble fibre as it is generally considered that this type of fibre reduces the risk of obesity, Type 2 Diabetes and also colon cancer.

In the case of Type 2 Diabetes, soluble fibre, because of its absorbent qualities, may control blood sugar by delaying gastric emptying, retarding the entry of glucose into the blood stream and lessening the post meal rise in blood sugar.

The cholesterol lowering effect of soluble fibres may also help in reducing heart disease risks. It appears that soluble fibre reduces cholesterol because of the gel it forms once mixed with water. As it passes through the digestive tract, the gel traps some substances related to high cholesterol.

There is an increasing amount of evidence that this process may lessen heart disease risks because of the reduced amount of cholesterol that is absorbed into the blood stream.

Studies find that people on high soluble fibre diets have lower total cholesterol levels and may be less likely to form harmful blood clots than those who consume low fibre diets.

A recent USA report found that, in sufficient amounts, fibre apparently reduced heart disease risks among men who ate more than 25 grams per day, compared to those consuming below 15 grams per day.

Just by changing the balance of your diet to eat more fresh vegetables and fruit will automatically give you more soluble fibre so this will not only help your bowels but your heart as well.

Soluble fibre is best

I got side-tracked on Type 2 Diabetes and high cholesterol but the benefits of soluble fibre over and above colon health are worth mentioning because often you will find that foods and diets that are good for the health of one part of the body are often good for other parts as well! A Mediterranean diet for example is good for both your heart and colon!

Soluble fibre, because it holds on to water, promotes greater cleansing. The gooey nature of soluble fibre actually helps absorb nasties and take them through to the bowel where they are eliminated.

Why we 'overdose' on wheat – the very fibre that may be making your constipation worse

So it is clear that we need more fibre, but it would appear that the one type of fibre that we rely on most is from wheat, and it is this type of fibre which can have the opposite effect to what you want.

This is because wheat can be mucus forming when taken to excess.

It's not only about the wheat you eat in your every-day foods such as bread and pasta, it is the hidden wheat that you get in prepared foods and pastries. You'll find it in the ingredients list in practically every prepared food you consume. It is very easy to 'overdose' on wheat without knowing it

This is why people who are trying to avoid wheat, particularly coeliacs, have such a difficult time adjusting to diets without wheat.

So, if wheat is such a major part of our diets and if, as many believe, it is a major contributor to our clogged and toxic systems, it's worth taking a closer look at.

Wheat – one of the main mucus forming culprits

Grains are the seeds of plants from the grass family which includes wheat, oats, barley, rye, maize, rice and millet. They are without doubt the most commonly consumed foods in the world – with wheat, maize and rice dominating worldwide consumption.

In the UK, wheat is a long established dietary staple, traditionally known to provide a good variety of vitamins and minerals, fibre and complex carbohydrates for lasting energy. Unfortunately the wheat which our ancestors knew and loved, would bear little resemblance to the wheat that fills the supermarket shelves today.

It is genetically selected to be hardy with a high gluten content (50% of protein content).

As a result the wheat we consume today is hard to digest and can irritate the intestinal tract. Gluten is a sticky molecule which traps air in the bread making process. Bakers use more gluten today because it makes the bread expand more and therefore increases its size. They have encouraged strains of wheat which contain higher levels of gluten so we are all being exposed to higher levels than normal.

Also, wheat is a cheap source of modified starch which is used to bulk out many commercial foods and this means you are probably eating more gluten than you think.

Gluten is the protein component in certain grains and is made up of insoluble glutanins and soluble gliadins. It is the gliadin that is mostly responsible for allergies and intolerance reactions. Gluten containing grains are: Wheat, spelt, rye, barley and oats. All of these contain gliadin except for oats.

Although gluten is a tough gelatinous substance that is hard to digest, most of us could cope with it if it wasn't consumed so widely. Because wheat is so prevalent, it can put a great strain on some systems. Roller milled wheat used for white bread is particularly hard to break down.

How can gluten become mucus forming?

There is a very simple answer to this question – because it is difficult to break down.

If your digestive system is weak and your production of stomach acid is low, protein can empty from the stomach without being properly broken down. This can put a strain on the small intestine which prefers to receive 'sludge' rather than small 'clumps'.

The small intestine may then see these 'clumps' as foreign bodies and as an act of self defence, surround them with protective mucus. Unfortunately, this mucus is not clear and slippery as would be produced in a healthy digestive system, it is cloudy, thick and sticky.

This sticky matter quickly dries out and can start to slow the digestive system down. This can then be the start of the whole process of 'clogging'.

In isolation this is not a problem but if this continues with the consumption of excessive amounts of wheat it is not difficult to see how things can start to go wrong and how people can start to build up intolerance to gluten.

Coeliac Disease or gluten allergy is a condition where gluten damages the delicate lining of the small intestine leading to malabsorption of nutrients and typically weight loss.

In the UK the condition affects 1 in 1000 and does seem to run in families. One theory is that coeliac disease is a manifestation of humans' inability to adapt to wheat. Coeliacs have to strictly avoid all gluten, although recent studies have shown that gliadin is the real culprit and that up to 80% of coelicas can in fact tolerate oats.

Gluten intolerance can also present problems in individuals who are not coeliac.

Wheat intolerance is rarely the cause of a true food allergy, but a frequent offender in food intolerance. Sometimes it is simply the fact that wheat is consumed so frequently and in such large volumes that causes the problem. Our diets are not as varied as they used to be and it is not difficult to see how our eating habits can be dictated by the large supermarkets.

It is difficult to find a prepared meal that does not contain some level of wheat.

Symptoms of wheat intolerance vary and often do not occur immediately after eating wheat-based foods. For this reason, people rarely connect their symptoms with food intolerance. If you eat wheat regularly and suffer from digestive complaints such as bloating or irritable bowel syndrome, mental and behavioural problems such as depression or hyperactivity, fatigue or headaches - it may be that you have developed an intolerance.

If you are wheat intolerant but continue to eat this grain on a regular basis, then digestive problems such as a clogged up system and leaky gut can arise.

A growing proportion of the population are now thought to suffer from leaky gut where the lining of the digestive tract has been damaged and becomes more permeable.

In the busy daily lives we lead, it is not difficult to see how wheat can be consumed in large quantities. You could have toast or wheat based cereal for breakfast, a sandwich or baguette for lunch and pasta or pizza for dinner ....it's easy to see how we can slip into the trap of eating wheat three times a day and that's not including the biscuits and snack bars in-between!

Young, single people are particularly vulnerable. It is not surprising that food intolerances appear to be increasing in our young people whose food choices tend to be much more limited than their parents.

When leaky gut has developed, gluten grains are not to be recommended because of the further irritation they can cause. In addition, because gluten is hard to digest it is more likely to pass through a leaky gut into the blood stream. The body will tag this gluten invader as foreign and mount an immune response.

So, if you are one of these people who consume more wheat because you want to get more fibre into your diet, you may in fact be causing your system to produce more mucus because of the over consumption of gluten and this, in time, could be worsening your constipation!

So wheat, a major part of the UK diet, can be a hidden contributor to the clogging of our digestive systems.

Unfortunately there is another food category that is a core part of the typical British diet which may also be clogging your digestive system (and arteries).

CHAPTER 6

Mucus forming foods and your constipation

Did you know the UK consumes more dairy produce per head than any other European country? Why do we consume so much? Is milk an essential source of calcium and protein or are we clogging up our systems with mucus forming matter?

What's the Problem?

The most common form of dairy intolerance is 'lactose intolerance' – this is when a person reacts to the milk sugar - lactose. Lactose malabsorption is common in those of African, Asian, Arabic and North American Indian descent as these races produce little or no lactase enzyme.

Why we smell funny to the Japanese

I was a regular visitor to Japan in the 1980's and after a few sakis would often get into deep discussions with my Japanese hosts. On one night when we were discussing the differences between Westerners and the Orientals, they started to snigger. As the Japanese hate to cause offence, it took me some time to squeeze it out of them, but they have this word for westerners which relates to our smell. Basically it means that we smell 'sour,' or of milk. Japanese people, like other Orientals do not consume dairy or if they do it is in very minute quantities. Because we, in the west, consume so much by comparison, it must 'ooze' through our skin. Clearly we do not notice it ourselves – it takes those who do not consume dairy to notice.

Lactose intolerance can develop in anyone. One of the main triggers for the development of milk intolerance is antibiotic use. Whilst doing their job of fighting infections antibiotics also kill off friendly bacteria which can help us to digest milk. So even if you have had no problem with milk in the past, you may find that, following antibiotics or a severe gastric upset, you show some of these typical malabsorption symptoms:

Abdominal bloating, diarrhoea, flatulence, malnutrition, nausea, abdominal cramps, foul smelling stools.

Symptoms typically occur 30 minutes to two hours after consumption of dairy foods but can also slowly develop over a longer period. You may also find that you can tolerate a small amount of lactose and it is only when the levels of dairy produce reach a certain threshold that you run into problems.

Dairy produce can be problematical for another reason. The protein in milk – casein - is difficult to digest and encourages mucus production. The following conditions have all been linked to dairy intake and have been known to show some improvement when dairy has been excluded from the diet;

Eczema, asthma, allergic colitis, arthritis, sinusitis, glue ear, migraine, hay fever.

People who are susceptible to mucus forming in their lungs such as asthma, are also more likely to be susceptible to mucus forming elsewhere including the gut.

Milk and dairy, along with wheat, are thought to be the most mucus forming products. Before looking at less mucus forming alternatives, let's just look at the effect of too much mucus in the body and discover why we must try to prevent it from building up and choking everything.

Why too much 'bad' mucus can contribute to your constipation

Throughout, I have made references to mucus forming foods that can be one of the causes of waste build up in the digestive tract. One of the primary advocates of this theory is Dr. Robert Gray, an American nutritionist.

In his booklet *The Colon Health Handbook*, he blames the consumption of too many mucus forming foods as being the main causes of colon disease and ultimately many of the common illnesses found in the West.

He determined, through intensive testing that certain foods are mucus forming and others are mucus cleansing. The foods shown to cause mucus are dairy products, white flour, meat, eggs, potatoes, beans, rice, grains, fish, peanuts and fats.

His views are pretty extreme and in my view, would be impossible for most of us to follow. In any case, foods like eggs and fish have so many health benefits they far outweigh any mucus problems they may cause.

It's all about finding the right balance. Eggs and fish are perfect, healthy foods and must make up part of your diet. However, if the rest of your diet is made up only of mucus forming foods, the benefits of taking healthy foods like eggs and fish will be lost.

To convert to a real cleansing diet will mean quite big adjustments for most of you, but once steps are taken, benefits will be felt very quickly, particularly with your digestive system. Your energy levels should improve as well.

So, it is obvious that some foods are more mucus forming than others. The secret to success is for you to cut out the worst offenders like wheat, dairy and red meat as much as you can, and then balance out other foods like fish, grains, beans and rice with lots of fresh vegetables, fruit and salad type foods.

The relationship between mucus and diet is not a new theory. In 1912, Dr. Arnold Ehret released a book called, *The Mucusless Diet and Healing System.* He discusses, in great detail, the mucus-forming effect of various foods. Ehret theorised that all disease is caused by a clogging of the tube and membrane structures within the body due to a build-up of restrictive mucus.

This theory has similarities to the Gerson Diet which encourages the use of high levels of organic vegetable and fruit juices (cleansing, non-mucus forming foods) to cleanse the body and rid it of many serious diseases including cancer.

To understand mucus in your body, if your body gets attacked with a cold virus then you know about it. You get a sore throat, puffy eyes and running nose.

In the same way your digestive system will react if it is consistently under attack from food it finds difficulty coping with. It will react by producing mucus.

High levels of mucus are a sure sign of a body in a state of extreme agitation. The heavy, over-processed, dairy-rich UK diet and the excess levels of wheat demand that the body reacts as if it is fighting a viral invasion every day.

Gray said that most people getting to middle age and beyond can feel its effect in the morning. Symptoms such as a foggy clogged head, puffy eyes and dulled senses are not uncommon. If you are intolerant to wheat and dairy then these symptoms will probably occur much earlier.

Candida, a fungal yeast overgrowth which establishes itself in the gut can be attributed to a weakened digestive system under great pressure from foods it finds difficult to digest. Candida itself can be totally debilitating and many practitioners theorise that ME and related diseases can be attributed to this overgrowth.

Clearly these types of symptoms can be attributed to any number of ailments, but if a clogged system is your problem, then you might be amazed at how a change in diet – one which is more in keeping with a cleansing diet - can improve how you feel within just a few weeks.

If we look at the human body a bit more closely, it is an incredibly complex system. It transfers vital fluids through miles of tubes and membrane highways. The circulatory system, apparently, is 60,000 miles long. The kidneys, alone, contain miles of internal plumbing.

However, mucus can slow down or stop the important movements along the many pathways of the body, creating a feeding ground for viruses and pathogens (disease-producing bacteria).

As mentioned earlier, not all mucus is bad. Healthy mucus is a clear, slippery, lubricating secretion, used to protect mucus membranes along the digestive, respiratory, urinary and reproductive tracts.

Unhealthy mucus is cloudy, thick, and sticky. It is secreted to stop irritants, pollutants, or carcinogenic compounds that are created by putrefying, undigested food residues. It's like a blanket of protection.

As we have seen already, certain foods such as milk and bread are particularly responsible for an increase of mucus secretions. These foods have large protein molecules (casein and gluten) which are difficult to digest, are more prone to putrefaction and may be toxic or irritating to the body. Also, for many, bread and milk cause sinus congestion.

Mucus is most commonly associated with the respiratory system when people get asthma. However, mucus is also very closely associated with the gastrointestinal tract, lymphatic system, uterus, urinary system and the joints.

Cartilage in a joint contains mucus membrane cells which secrete a clear slippery mucus to keep joints lubricated. When mucus-forming substances are produced in the digestive tract as a reaction to food irritants, this toxic mucoid build up could eventually find its way and deposit itself within your joints.

This can be particularly true if your gut becomes 'leaky' or permeable after years of erosion by mucus forming foods or too much consumption of non-steroidal anti-inflammatories, asprin, alcohol and other pollutants.

Many cases of inflammation of the joints can be traced back to problems in the guts.

This is why looking at your bowel health might be a good starting point for inflammation in your joints!

Why chewing your food more thoroughly will help reduce your constipation and improve your overall health

Chewing food thoroughly and slowly will reduce the effects of intolerance, and help you absorb more nutrients from your food. This means that less 'bad' mucus is produced and less clogging of your digestive tract. In turn this will reduce your chances of constipation and give you better general health. It doesn't cost you anything, so you should focus more on it.

Also, as a bonus, if you are trying to lose weight, chewing your food thoroughly and more slowly will give more time for your stomach to send signals to your brain that you are full, and this will help you to eat less and to avoid over-eating.

Foods that form mucus have a glue-like bond, tightly holding their molecules together. As a reminder, in milk it is casein and in wheat, rye, oats and barley, the glue-like substance is gluten. The dictionary defines gluten as a tough, sticky mixture of plant proteins, obtained by washing out the starch from wheat or other cereal flour and used as an adhesive and thickener. These glue-like bonds require strong stomach acids for digestion.

So, if you don't chew your food properly, eat too many mucus forming foods and not enough cleansing foods and have low stomach acid, it is highly likely that you are in the fast lane for congestion resulting ultimately in constipation.

Lack of chewing and poor food combinations make it impossible for the stomach acids to properly dissolve the bond between these molecules. After digestion, many food particles are still too large to be used by the body. In a short time, the oversized, partly-digested food particles start to putrefy and are coated with mucus to prevent further putrefaction while still in the intestine.

As the mucus and food particle solution pass through the intestines, moisture is removed. As more moisture is removed, the mucus becomes sticky and gluey. Gray and Ehert believed that this can leave a coating on the intestinal wall.

Robert Gray indicated that layer after layer of gluey waste matter builds up over the years. It forms into lumps of a tough, rubbery, black substance in the corners of the intestinal tract. According to reports I have read, X-ray studies show that the accumulation of hardened faeces badly deforms the intestines.

Autopsies have shown that an average male has between seven and nine pounds of hardened faeces within his intestine. This coating causes constipation, a reduction in the absorption of nutrients through the intestinal wall and is a breeding ground for parasites.

And so we move on to the colon. If waste matter going from the small intestine is gluey and sticky it will quickly dry the colon out. The longer it hangs around in the colon, the drier the stools become until they are difficult to pass. The hardness can then push outwards and downwards causing a strain on the system and leading to problems like diverticular disease (where small pockets form in the colon wall) and haemorrhoids, where downward pressure on the rectum area pushes veins out.

A clogged up colon is a bit like a drain clogged with human hair, dust, old soap and pieces of decaying food, all forming a sticky mass of rotting waste that cannot be removed.

Different foods putrefy at different speeds.

The tendency of a food to putrefy or spoil in the body is parallel to that of the same food outside the body. If you let fresh fruit sit outside the fridge, it usually takes several days before it begins to spoil. At the same temperature, fresh vegetables will usually spoil in less time than fresh fruit.

On the other hand, unrefrigerated raw meat will spoil in less than a day's time. Moreover, cooking any food generally causes it to spoil quicker than it would if left raw.

Because the temperature inside the digestive tract is in the vicinity of 38 degrees centigrade, putrefaction of food within the body takes place much more rapidly than at room temperature.

Those foods that putrefy quickly, such as meat, fish, eggs and pasteurised dairy products, are more difficult to digest, so may go through to the colon more slowly anyway. Vegetables and fruits on the other hand are easily digested and therefore they have very little putrefactive impact, if any, compared to meat and dairy.

This is why it is so important to keep waste matter moving along. Going to the loo every two or three days is not sufficient – particularly if your diet is made up primarily by mucus forming foods.

Some pointers to help prevent your digestive system getting clogged up

• Eat small meals

Our body's need for food is often much less than what we eat. Any foods eaten beyond our body's need is a burden. Some of this excess food will be converted into fat. Yet the body can create only so much fat per day. If you eat above digestive capacity, the excess must be eliminated. During elimination, the lymph glands are overloaded and mucoid forms in response to putrefaction

• Eat only when hungry

When food is eaten before complete digestion of the previous meal, partially-digested food will be released into the colon thus causing mucus.

• Don't gulp your food

Improper chewing overworks the digestive system. If the food particles are too big to be assimilated, they must be eliminated through the colon. On the way, these particles putrefy, thus causing mucus.

• Avoid low levels of zinc

Levels of stomach acid decline with age. If the levels of stomach acid are too low, protein is not broken down properly in the stomach and this can mean undigested food particles entering the small intestine, leading to putrefaction and an increase in mucus. Low levels of stomach acid are related to low zinc levels as it is this mineral which is most important for acid production in the stomach. Also acid in the stomach is the means by which the many foes such as viruses, bacteria, yeast and parasites are killed off. Low acid gives bad breath. Health department figures show that 31 percent of men and women get less than the recommended dietary intake for zinc, so this is something everyone should consider over the age of 40.

• Things to avoid (if possible)

Antibiotics, stress, refined sugar, alcohol, long term use of non-steroidal anti-inflammatories (NSAIDs). All of these can change the mucous lining of the intestines.

Now we know more about the potential causes of a build up of mucus in your system, the next stage is to look at the consequences of this.

CHAPTER 7

The implications of Impacted waste

A sluggish, congested, digestive system can also put pressure on other parts of the elimination system.

Your bowels are just one part of the sophisticated waste disposal system in your body. If your bowels themselves are not eliminating properly this can put added strain on other parts of the body that are there to cleanse the body of unwanted waste. The liver, kidneys, lungs, digestive system, lymphatic system and skin can all be considered to be important parts of this disposal system.

An increasing toxic load from our environment and an increasing level of drugs and chemical additives in our diets means that our waste removal system is having to work ever harder.

Your liver and kidneys need to function efficiently if your digestive system is to be cleansed

Your liver is a particularly important organ because it helps to break down your chemical waste and transport it to the digestive system. Reducing red meat and dairy protein and saturated fat will help your liver function better. Alcohol, NSAIDs (Non Steroidal Anti-Inflammatory Drugs) and chemicals in food can put extra strain on your liver so avoiding these as far as possible is important.

Your kidneys need plenty of water to function properly. Cranberry juice, cucumbers and melons are good for kidney health as are leeks, onions, celery and garlic, so increase these and reduce refined sugar and salt which are not good.

I have mentioned the Gerson Diet a couple of times in this book. The Gerson therapy uses copious amounts of pure juices and foods to help the body to recover from serious illnesses. One of their soup recipes, called Hippocrates Soup, is recommended daily as a tonic for the kidneys. This is comprised of leeks, tomatoes, onions, garlic, potatoes and celery. You simply make a soup with nothing added.

The lymphatic system - another important part of the elimination factory

One of the major roles of the lymphatic system is to remove toxins from your body. It does this through a series of channels around your body which are similar to veins and arteries. The channels are filled with a fluid called lymph that circulates the body in one direction. This fluid acts as a carrier for dead cells and unwanted waste matter, which are ultimately eliminated via the lymph nodes. The lymphatic system does not have a pump like the heart to circulate the fluid, so its efficiency depends on your lifestyle.

Skin brushing and massage are effective ways of improving lymph drainage.

Your bowels do not work in isolation

It is important to emphasise the role that different parts of the elimination system play so that you can understand that your bowels do not work in isolation and that, in fact, they play a part in a very intricate waste disposal system. Your bowels play an extremely important role in both the digestive and elimination systems in your body and for this reason your bowel function should not be treated in isolation with a 'quick fix'.

A clogged up bowel does not only affect the bowel itself with problems such as diverticular disease, it also impacts on other parts of the elimination and digestive systems. So, how your digestive system functions further up can influence how your bowel functions over time and vice versa.

A constipated bowel therefore impacts the health of your whole body. Below are some terms that you may come across which make reference to the consequences of impacted waste.

Autointoxication

This is the process whereby the body literally poisons itself by maintaining a cesspool of decaying matter in its colon. As we have seen earlier, if decaying matter is not expelled efficiently then harmful bacteria will take a hold and the resulting toxins can get into the bloodstream and travel to all parts of the body. Autointoxication can be the catalyst for many diseases.

Putrefaction

This is the process of the decay of food in the digestive system. In a healthy bowel, putrefaction hardly takes place at all. But in a sluggish bowel where waste matter has been hanging around for too long - putrefaction occurs. How bad this gets depends on the type of diet, how sluggish the system is and the efficiency of the digestive and elimination systems.

Stagnation

This is the failure of the digestive tract and bowels to expel waste matter efficiently. Stagnation occurs primarily in the colon and is usually the body's main contributor to putrefaction and the consequent autointoxication.

The longer waste matter hangs around, the more likely it is to putrefy. The average time in our western civilisation is 65 – 100 hours. It should be no longer than 24-36 hours.

The stagnant material in the colon can be divided into two types - putrefactive and post-putrefactive. The former is still moist, decaying, and releasing toxic substances. Unless it is removed it eventually becomes so dry and hard that it doesn't putrefy any further. It then becomes post-putrefactive and is very difficult to dissolve or remove.

It is known that parasites thrive upon stagnant putrefactive matter within the intestines.

Diarrhoea – one of the unlikely consequences of a toxic colon

There are many thousands of people who suffer chronic diarrhoea. If you are one of these people and have been checked out by your doctor and found that there is no obvious disease then the next few lines are for you.

For starters, you must not rule out the fact that your diarrhoea is in fact the result of many years of constipation or at least many years of a diet high in mucus foods and low in cleansing foods.

There may have been other things going on. Problems might have been exacerbated by poor digestion, inflammatory bowel disease, food allergies, intestinal parasites, candidiasis to name but a few.

All of these could be related to long term constipation. Clearly there can be many other factors such as stress, but it doesn't require a lot of imagination to understand that long term constipation can certainly make things much worse.

Very few people connect diarrhoea to past constipation. Why should they? Constipation and diarrhoea are often seen as being opposite ends of the pole. However, if loose stools are caused by a toxic colon, there is a term for it; it is known as 'inadequate contact diarrhoea'. This actually means that your diarrhoea might in fact be a form of constipation, caused by a clogged colon.

Remember that one of the jobs of the colon is to reabsorb water from the liquid waste matter that arrives from the small intestine. This enables stools to be formed ready for evacuation.

If however, this liquid waste matter cannot get into contact with the colon wall because it is encrusted with decaying waste, the water cannot be reabsorbed and stools cannot be formed. The liquid waste matter then just skids straight through.

You then get into a 'Catch 22' situation. If things move too fast then the all important healthy bacteria also flashes by. Good bacteria needs a stable and moist environment to establish itself, not the type of environment where diarrhoea is present. Until the system slows down it is virtually impossible to re-establish the all-important good bacteria.

The best natural product I know for slowing down the digestive system naturally is the fibre, psyllium husk. I will talk more about this in Chapter 10. Psyllium husk helps to consolidate matter naturally giving any good bacteria in the system some time to get established and to start fighting the bad guys.

A colon that is without good bacteria leaves itself open to putrefaction and impacted waste. Maintaining the levels of good bacteria is therefore absolutely crucial in the battle of keeping your colon 'clean'.

In cases of diarrhoea, psyllium husk can be a great asset in the armoury to break the cycle and to start getting things back to normal. Psyllium is also very effective at gradually clearing away old waste matter.

Are your guts leaking?

Clearly a digestive tract that has accumulated toxic waste over the years has the potential to become 'stressed' and irritated. I referred to leaky gut earlier on but it is worth elaborating on it a bit more as it is so often the consequence of a colon that is under attack.

The digestive system is a long tube, the lining of which is only one cell thick; this lining is called the mucosal barrier. Your digestive tract wall is supposed to act as a barrier between the sludge of broken down food that is passing through your digestive tract and your bloodstream, only letting through those nanoparticles of food that your body needs for good health. The remainder of the sludge, not required by the body, moves on to the large colon.

There is a tight junction between adjacent cells which constitutes this barrier. However, when the lining becomes infected or inflamed this barrier becomes loose, allowing large molecules such as undigested or partly digested food, bacteria, fungi and toxic chemicals to pass through. When these foreign substances enter the bloodstream they can trigger an immune response.

Medication such as antibiotics and NSAIDs can make the situation worse. Antibiotics are well known for killing bad bacteria. Unfortunately, they don't differentiate between good and bad bacteria in your digestive tract, particularly in your large bowel. The good bacteria form a protective shield on the walls of your digestive system and if they are knocked out by the antibiotics, your gut wall can be weakened.

Another attack to your system can come from the widely prescribed NSAID's which have a habit of punching holes in your digestive tract. Excessive alcohol can have the same effect.

As we have seen already, reactions or intolerances to certain foods can also cause stress. The obvious examples being wheat and dairy but there are many others. Undigested food floating around and decaying in the gut can provide the perfect conditions for irritating the intestinal wall, making it 'leaky.'

It doesn't require much imagination to understand that allowing toxic waste into the bloodstream cannot be good for health. For this reason many practitioners believe that all, if not most, disease starts with a toxic colon which leaks waste matter which should otherwise be eliminated.

Symptoms of a Leaky Gut

These can be summarised as: Bloating, chronic fatigue, Irritable Bowel Syndrome, increased susceptibility to viruses and bacterial infections, poor digestion, sensitivity to a range of foods, weakened immunity and inflammatory responses in your joints such as arthritis.

Leaky Gut Syndrome is associated with a range of medical problems, including food allergies, Coeliac disease and Crohn's disease. It is also linked to a number of auto-immune diseases such as asthma, atopy, eczema, psoriasis, and rheumatoid arthritis. Interestingly, childhood autism is strongly associated with leaky gut syndrome.

Should you have inflammation in your joints, investigating the health and efficiency of your colon should be the first move before reaching for your glucosamine or anti-inflammatory drugs.

Finding the cause usually means finding the answer.

The importance of glutamine

In Chapter 9 I talk about certain nutrients that are very important to the health of your digestive tract. The most important is the amino acid known as glutamine. This nutrient is in every cell that lines your digestive tract but it can get depleted very easily when you and your digestive system are under stress.

Without it, your digestive tract cannot maintain its normal barrier qualities so I would recommend that everyone with leaky gut or looking to improve overall bowel and digestive tract health should take this nutrient. It is widely available as a powder or in capsules. Many athletes take it as it is considered so important for the immune system.

A toxic colon, bad breath and body odour

Whereas it might seem logical that a toxic colon cannot be good for our overall health if it continues unabated, there are other unpleasant consequences that could affect you on the way. It could make your stools smell too strong and give you bad breath.

Young girls in particular can be prone to the beginnings of a congested digestive system when they go on their low fat, low calorie diets.

As maintaining a healthy weight is not only good for our health but also our vanity, I have devoted a separate chapter on your digestive system and its role in keeping you nice and slim.

Yes, you guessed it, you cannot lose weight healthily or effectively with a toxic colon.

CHAPTER 8

You can't lose weight when you are constipated

This statement puts forward the theory that if your digestive system is not effective then you can't lose weight efficiently and healthily. In other words having decaying waste matter hanging around in the colon which should otherwise be eliminated is not conducive to getting good results when you stand on the scales in the morning.

Being overweight is a sign that your body is under stress and it is highly likely that a sluggish digestive system – and the wrong choice of 'dead' foods has played a part.

A constipated system means that more toxic waste is hanging around and getting into the bloodstream putting greater strain on the liver and lymphatic systems in particular. If the body is unable to get rid of waste effectively, it will dump them in fat cells to keep them out of harm's way.

This dumped body waste is better known as cellulite which everyone knows is difficult to get rid of. This is because the body is reluctant to release unwanted toxins back into a system that is not eliminating properly. It goes without saying that if your bowels are eliminating effectively then this reduces pressure on other parts of the waste disposal system and gives you a greater chance of reducing cellulite.

A constipated system is highly acidic. Making the system more alkaline by eating more cleansing fruits and vegetables will give you far greater chance of reducing and eliminating cellulite. I will be talking more about your acid/alkaline balance in Chapter 9.

Protein and grains are acid forming foods. This doesn't mean that you should stop eating protein and grains. On the contrary, they are a necessary part of your diet. If your intake of fresh vegetables, fruit and salad foods exceed the intake of proteins and grains throughout the day then you are more likely to be in an alkaline state and this will, in turn, reduce constipation, make you feel better and make it easier for you to lose weight.

A healthy digestive system has to be good for your weight and ultimately your health.

The typical low fat diet can be one of the causes of mucus forming foods that are likely to clog up your system.

Some estimates suggest that even young people could be holding on to as much as 15lbs of excess waste matter in their bowels and this could be equivalent to seven bags of sugar! This is probably due to the popularity of fast food these days.

I find that many diets (particularly the high protein diets) can make you very constipated very quickly and this doesn't make sense if you are trying to lose weight. But no matter what type of diet you are on, you should be looking more towards reducing mucus forming foods in your diet and increasing the cleansing ones if you want to lose weight sensibly and healthily.

Low fat yoghurts contain high percentages of dairy and the low fat convenient foods that a large number of people go for inevitably contain wheat in some form.

The fad for high meat protein diets can, in my view, be particularly dangerous. They can increase the potential for putrefaction and lead to waste matter being reabsorbed into your blood causing skin problems, bad breath, body odour and weight gain.

The last things you want if you are trying to look good!

The reality is that food should not remain in your system for more than 24 hours after eating. Imagine how unhygienic and disgusting your kitchen would be if you did not empty your bin regularly and kept bags of rotting rubbish around for days and weeks. It is no different with your colon!

Over the last 20 years we have been told to eat more fibre. As it is drummed into us day-in and day-out, you would have thought it would have been quite easy for every one to achieve this. In the 1980's high fibre diets to help weight-loss were in vogue. These days it's more about low fat.

The low fat diet has been a fad for many years and you would assume that by removing fat you would leave more room for fibre. Sadly this is not true. The fat has just been replaced by more carbohydrates and refined sugar. In most cases, it hasn't been replaced by fresh fruit and vegetables, the foods you really need to keep your digestive system working properly and your weight under control.

It's not easy to lose weight if your digestive system is only working at 50%! The waste that hangs around in your system is literally 'dead weight' and needs to be cleared away.

If you can cleanse your colon with the right balance of cleansing foods this will help you lose weight and make you feel better and cleaner both inside and out! Your skin is likely to become clearer and your breath fresher too!

Why your new cleansing diet is good for your Body Mass Index (BMI) and weight loss

More research is showing that a diet with a high percentage of fibre is conducive to losing weight. This fits in nicely with a diet that is high in cleansing foods which will be naturally high in fibre anyway.

One example of some recent research was from Tufts University in the US. In the research it was found that in the case of women in particular, those with low levels of fibre in their diet were far more likely to be overweight. Obesity was measured by the BMI.

It was found that there was a direct correlation between fibre intake and BMI. The higher the levels of fibre, the lower the BMI. Also, having more fibre in your diet was found to lower the glycaemic index of food, and this helps to slow the release of carbohydrates into the blood stream.

Your new diet will be helping you achieve healthy BMI levels by providing lots of naturally occurring fibre.

Body odour can indicate a toxic colon

There is a close relationship between body odour and putrefaction with the intestinal tract. So, you spend all this time to look good by losing weight and you then go and spoil it all with bad BO!

Overall body perspiration, with the possible exception of underarm perspiration, should not create a body odour problem if you bathe regularly. If you are unable to control overall body odour no matter how frequently you bathe this can often be down to a highly putrefactive colon.

A good indicator of intestinal putrefaction is foot odour. Your feet should not have a strong odour. If after wearing a pair of socks for just one day they become very smelly then it might be you have a putrefactive colon. Underarm smell is different. This is the one part of your body that you still have to deodorise, even after the colon is cleansed.

Hang around horrors – the foods that love to stay with you!

Throughout this book I have made references to stagnant waste matter hanging around causing problems.

This next bit of text came from a female magazine talking about bowel health. I thought it summarised quite nicely much of what I have been saying!!

Most people don't give their food a second thought once they've eaten it. You might pay more attention if you thought a meal could give you BO, bad breath and potentially cause a host of serious health problems.

What does an unhealthy diet really mean and what are its effects? Unhealthy food is so difficult for our bodies to digest it can hang round inside for weeks - sometimes as long as two months - simply rotting away, releasing toxins into our blood stream and encouraging parasites to thrive.

The top offenders are:

- *Fast-food burgers*
- *Mass production white bread*
- *Any pie made with pastry*
- *Ready meals*
- *Processed cheese*
- *Fast-food thick milk shakes*
- *Crisps*

So a diet of fast food cheese burgers with fries and a shake is the equivalent of eating yourself ill!

The toxins released by the decaying process get into the blood stream and travel to every part of the body. Each cell can then be affected, weakening the entire system and potentially being a factor in nearly any disease from obvious issues like haemorrhoids, to colon cancer, diverticulitis and even heart disease.

As time goes by, your colon gets increasingly toxic and works at half the capacity. When your digestive system is only working at 50%, it means your body is taking in a lot less of the goodness from your food and can even cause you to put on weight. The waste that hangs around in your system is literally 'dead weight' and needs to be cleared away.

Weight loss is a pleasant side effect of a healthy digestive system.

One of the side effects of cleansing your system and changing it from a 'stagnant, muddy stream' to one that is flowing freely with sparkling clean water, is that you will lose weight naturally. Not only will you lose weight naturally but it will happen without you having to calorie count.

By changing the balance of your diet, there is no necessity to starve yourself. In fact you don't have to go hungry at all.

As I have emphasised so much in this book, an efficient digestive system which expels waste matter efficiently will help you lose weight naturally. If you recall, I also mentioned that chewing your food well will get the whole digestive process off to a good start and therefore help you lose those pounds.

<u>Eating more slowly and chewing more efficiently will mean that you will feel full after eating less food.</u>

All you need do is to make sure that you have plenty of the more cleansing food and snacks around you for times when you might be tempted or you get hungry.

You've probably guessed by now that I am not a fan of the low fat diets that many people go on. Because these foods have little or no fibre it is not long before the digestive system slows down and constipation sets in. You may lose weight on a low calorie diet for two weeks or so but once this happens your body goes into 'survival' mode which is something our bodies have developed over thousands and thousands of years as a protection mechanism.

Your brain then starts telling you to eat more to make up for the lack of calorie intake.

If you are on a low fat diet, there is little to slow down the absorption of sugar into the bloodstream. The yoyo effect of high and low sugar then ensues and cravings start.

Low and behold, the diet comes to an abrupt end with little or no weight loss. If you have ever been on this type of diet in the past I am sure that, over time, you managed to put back on more weight than you struggled to lose in the first place.

However, the good news is that if you can follow a diet that removes the worst offending culprits of mucus, to one that is more cleansing, then blood sugars will automatically start to stabilise and the cravings can stop and you can lose weight, gradually but steadily, without having to worry about putting it back on.

Also you will find that those headaches that suddenly appeared when you started the low fat diets will suddenly disappear!

Wheat consumption, particularly if you are intolerant to it, can be one of the major causes of blood sugar swings and this is why you can lose a significant amount of weight (and feel much better) simply by taking wheat out of your diet. In fact any type of food intolerance can be related to sugar imbalances and cravings, so avoidance of the products most likely to cause digestive problems would be extremely helpful.

I am sure that just by thinking about trying to lose weight you get depressed. It's such hard work. Most diets are based on calorie counting, going hungry and avoiding the basic influence that prevents people from losing weight in the first place. That is, they ignore the fact that products that many people are intolerant to, such as wheat and dairy, can cause reactions in the body resulting in low blood sugar. This then leads to cravings and so it goes on. This is why you often crave the food you are intolerant to.

So you can forget all about calories and going hungry if you pursue a diet that helps to cleanse your digestive system. If you have an efficient and cleansed digestive system, you will automatically get to what your weight should be in the first place. So there is no need to keep getting on the scales. Instead, at your own pace, start changing the balance of your diet until you are getting it mainly right. This diet does not mean hardship. It just means finding tasty alternatives and getting plenty of them!

There are many basic processes that govern the way the body uses energy and burns up fat. If you can give it the right conditions with the right food, then your body will do this more efficiently. So more of the right food will automatically mean less body fat!!

What we are talking about here is better health, better weight, better well-being and more vitality and energy.

What is crucial to you losing weight is the removal of foods that fight the efficient workings of your body

This ironically does not mean the reduction of all fats. Some fats are good and will help your body be more efficient and healthy and this is covered in more detail in Chapter 10.

We all know that reducing calories one week and going back to normal the next just doesn't work. What I am suggesting in this book is that you change your diet, at your own speed, to one that is less mucus forming. It is not a quick fix but a long term commitment. As time goes on, this process will get easier because you will get to know the dos and don'ts and what you like and dislike.

The main point is that once you have redressed the balance of your diet and found that you need not go hungry, you will get to the weight you should be without thinking about it. So the secret to success is to take a long term view of your new diet. You are not going to get it right immediately but take time to find alternative foods that you like and introduce them as and when you can.

If you forget about losing weight but focus on a healthy diet then things will work for you. Look upon the weight loss as a bonus.

Flush those pounds away

If your body is dehydrated, then it will be far more difficult for you to lose weight. In the same way water is needed to flush toxins through the digestive tract, plenty of water will aid weight loss. The more flushing that goes on, the easier your body will be able to eliminate unwanted matter from your body.

Sometimes I hear of people cutting down their water intake when they have water retention. However, water retention is quite often a sign that you are dehydrated and that you need more water to flush things through.

Also, fluid retention can quite often be a sign of wheat intolerance.

Even a mild intolerance to wheat can affect the body by increasing the permeability of the capillaries which means that extra fluid flows into the cells. Abdominal bloating may be due to fluid retention or the digestive system not dealing with a particular food so well. Removing wheat usually removes bloating.

Why many detox diets make you feel 'rough.'

So, as I mentioned in the last chapter if you are changing your diet to one that is more cleansing than mucus forming, you will immediately be helping your eliminatory organs – the liver, kidneys, lungs, digestive tract and lymphatic systems to remove toxins. The more efficient they are – the more easily you will be able to lose weight.

As you start losing weight on your new diet, toxins that have been stored in fat tissue will gradually be released into the blood stream and this can make your feel rough for a while. This is because the waste, toxic matter is very acidic and your blood likes things that are more alkaline.

During this time it is absolutely vital that your bowels, along with your other eliminatory organs, are working efficiently so that the extra waste being released can be eliminated effectively and doesn't get reabsorbed.

If your eliminatory system is not working at full capacity when extra toxins are being released into your blood stream then you can expect some negative reactions like nausea and headaches.

Anything you can do at this time to remove acidic things in your diet will not only make you feel better, they will also help you to lose weight. This means removing or cutting back on wheat, meat proteins and some grains and increasing alkaline foods such as – you guessed it, - lots of fresh vegetables, fruits and salad. Remember to drink lots of water.

Avoid the tiredness often associated with low fat diets. Your new cleansing diet will stabilise your blood sugar balance.

Your blood sugars should be better balanced with your new cleansing diet so this is yet another way in which your new way of eating can help you to be trimmer. I mentioned earlier in this chapter that blood sugar imbalances hamper weight loss. As this is such an important issue, I believe it is worth looking into further.

By removing or reducing many of the main culprits of the mucus forming diet, your blood sugars will automatically become more stable. Unstable blood sugar can be one of the causes of cravings that send you right back to the biscuit tin. If you have ever tried a low calorie diet you will know what I mean. Most low calorie diets cut out fats. Unfortunately there are those fats which are essential (hence called the essential fatty acids) which, if removed from your diet, can have a destabilising effect on blood sugar.

This is because most low calorie diets contain a lot of carbohydrates and sugar which enters the blood stream far too quickly and some of this sugar is transferred to the muscles as fat. This overloads the blood with sugar and as a reaction to this, the pancreas, in-turn, over-reacts and produces too much insulin to get rid of the excess sugar. As a result, the blood sugar drops too low. This then can set off cravings for sweet foods and wheat based products like biscuits, bread and pasta.

This is where your diet and weight loss goes out of the window. It is known as the 'yoyo' effect. So, this is yet another reason for getting rid of wheat from your diet.

If you follow your new diet closely, this will have the effect of slowing down the absorption of sugar from carbohydrates in your meal. The carbohydrate in fruit, vegetables, beans, chickpeas and pulses etc is slow releasing so will not set off this 'yoyo' effect.

If you do get blood sugar swings, then it is a good idea to have a small amount of protein at most meals. Even if you are eating an apple, taking a few almonds just afterwards can slow sugar absorption down and keep things more stable. The level of protein you need however is small – no more than 15-20% intake. Peanuts are fine from time to time, but try and focus more on almonds, walnuts and brazil nuts.

Ways to keep your blood sugar stable

These include not skipping breakfast – ensure you have a substantial breakfast of say, a wheat free muesli with live yoghurt, followed by some raw peppers or some grilled fish occasionally. This is a typical type of the continental diet. Don't worry if you are breaking the mould of what you might normally have for breakfast.

One great tasty tip for breakfast is to have raw organic porridge with some pumpkin or sunflower seeds. If you have invested in a juicer, you can juice apples and use this to replace milk. It tastes great and it's really healthy for you.

Overall, keeping your blood sugar stable means eating little and often and that includes having some well balanced snacks during the day. These might include fruit and some nuts to eat twice a day when peckish.

Have a good lunch of salad and fresh vegetables with a small amount of beans or nuts with one of your three weekly portions of fish.

Eat a small, balanced evening meal. Eat enough to fill your stomach and no more. You will find just by cutting down on your evening intake will help you lose weight. If you are going out for a meal to a restaurant, it is easy to eat well and not overdo it. Avoid any bread, puddings and coffee and see how much more you enjoy your main meal!

For women it is particularly important to eat well in around the time of your period as you can become more vulnerable to blood sugar swings at this time.

Don't get depressed

Our moods can be influenced by serotonin, a neurotransmitter which is a chemical messenger present in the blood stream. If you can keep your serotonin levels up then the likelihood is that you will feel better – your mood will be lifted.

Eating fish, particularly oily fish like salmon, mackerel and herrings is particularly good for this. In addition to increasing serotonin levels, the active ingredients in fish, (EPA) have been shown to relieve depression.

If after a while of following the cleansing diet you do feel a little low, then your essential fatty intake might be a bit low. In this case there are two recommendations I can make.

The first is to increase your essential fatty acid intake by taking two teaspoons of organic flaxseed oil per day.

The second is to take a purified omega 3 supplement which contains at least 500mg of EPA per capsule.

Both of these supplements are in keeping with your new cleansing diet.

I stress that you take a purified form of Omega 3 fish oil as this is the best way to be sure the oil is not contaminated by pollutants. A purified fish oil is usually differentiated from other Omega 3 fish oils by the letters E-EPA on the front of the jar or box. This is vitally important because many people who lose weight and reduce fat in their diet also remove the good fat which includes the essential fatty acids like Omega 3 which has this all-important EPA. As a consequence to this, you can get mood swings and ultimately a depressed feeling - so what do you do? You go out and eat comfort foods and gain weight again.

So, certain types of fats are good for your health and – would you believe it – your weight as well. I want to look at this more closely in Chapter 10.

When I started this book, I did not envisage writing a complete chapter on weight loss. However it is absolutely clear to me that our obesity and constipation issues are indelibly linked. Too much mucus in our systems clogs up all our body's pathways including our elimination systems. Common sense would suggest that this is not conducive to healthy body weight.

So far I have looked at groups of foods that can have a cleansing and clogging effect. Let's now take a closer look at some specific choices that might help the new diet and some of those that won't.

CHAPTER 9

Some dietary recommendations to cleanse your digestive system and reduce mucus forming foods from your diet

Changing the balance of your diet from one which is mucus forming to one which is more mucus 'cleansing' isn't rocket science but at the same time it isn't easy to change old habits. If you rush at this, you may get fed up too quickly, so the main idea is to give yourself a reasonable time scale to move the pendulum in the other direction.

At the end of this chapter I have listed some alternative options to the most common types of foods to avoid. But first and foremost, remember to keep yourself hydrated – this will be a vital part of your cleansing process.

Water, water and more water

The most important thing you need to survive is oxygen. The second is water. It makes up 70% of your body and you can't live long without it. It's easy however to get dehydrated and to underestimate what you need to drink daily to keep fit and healthy.

Lots of water is vital to bowel health and most of us do not drink enough of it. The more water going through, the better the 'flush' effect you get in your system. Plenty of water can help to reduce the mucus effect and slow down the 'drying' process.

Just how much extra water you need is always difficult to pin down but aim for a minimum of two litres per day on top of your normal intake.

Drinking a pint first thing in the morning is a good start to the day. Add a twist of lemon or some squeezed grapefruit and this can help give your liver a boost. Otherwise the best advice is to drink little and often throughout the day.

Initially taking in extra liquid can be a burden but if you organise yourself properly then you can make sure that water is always available.

If you don't like the taste of tap water then you can consider having a filter put on your tap. They can be expensive and may need servicing once per year but, overall, they are cheaper than bottled water and more convenient.

To my mind this investment is well worth it. In my experience many people react (without knowing it) to tap water, particularly in those areas where fluoride is added. Also, a good filtering system will remove this and other contaminants such as excess lead. The purer the water the better the cleansing effect, this is why I recommend a good filtering system if you can afford it. There is also growing evidence that some water packed in plastic bottles is not quite as pure as it should be.

A successful 'cleansing' diet will mean quite a substantial increase in soluble fibre and this, in turn, needs lots of water if it is going to give you the benefits you need.

Remember not to count tea or coffee in your drink intake because they can be dehydrating in themselves.

The best time for drinking extra liquid is around 30 minutes before a meal and then anytime in the day but not immediately after a meal. Generally I recommend not drinking for around 30 minutes after a meal. This includes coffee. Drinking too much during a meal can sometimes dilute digestive enzyme activity and therefore impede digestion.

Of course be sensible about this. If your meal is dry you can drink small amounts of liquid such as water or juice but don't overdo it. Wine should always be in moderation.

I often see young people not chewing their food properly, washing everything down with copious amounts of cola. This is a recipe for disaster in the long term. If their diet is not good in the first place with lots of white bread, burgers and dairy then you can start to see the development of food intolerances and the early onset of digestive and bowel problems.

Dilute your fruit juices

Many juices are made from concentrate and therefore have high levels of fruit sugar. Perhaps the best way to consume these types of drinks is to dilute with water 50/50. Smoothies are better because they incorporate the whole fruit. Adding wheat grass or some recommended green juice powder from your local health shop will add to the 'cleansing' effect. Once you get used to pure, natural juices you will find the packaged fruit concentrates too sweet.

Limit your tea and coffee intake

As a general rule, keep tea and coffee to no more than three cups per day. The caffeine present in tea and coffee can have a dehydrating effect when consumed to excess and this will fight your cleansing programme.

There are literally so many alternatives these days, with a bit of effort and experimentation you will find something that suits.

I've always been a tea man and used to consume between four to five cups per day. Over the last five years I have been working to reduce my dairy intake. Up until twelve months ago I had achieved 95% success – the only bit that eluded me was the milk that I had in tea. I was convinced that no matter what, this is something that I could not live without.

However, I made sure that at work in particular, I had a variety of herbal teas to try so that throughout the day I could try different types in between my normal tea. Very gradually I found that I wasn't missing my tea with milk. My favourite tipples now are organic green tea and peppermint tea with liquorice tea thrown in as a change every now and again. In fact when I do go back to my normal tea I am finding it rather bland with the milk giving it a sour, 'dead' taste.

I do recall enjoying green tea when I visited Japan a few times in the 1980's but didn't continue taking it when returning to the UK. The great thing about such a drink is that it is a very powerful antioxidant – which means it helps with the cleansing process – and it is increasingly linked with protection against certain types of cancer, including cancer of the Prostate – so it's nice to enjoy a drink knowing that it is helping to cleanse your system at the same time!

When overseas I tend to drink coffee rather than tea. Like most people I love a cappuccino but found that this was definitely out of bounds if I was to really progress with my dairy free diet. Your local health store will offer you lots of coffee alternatives but overall, if you are like me, you will find the herbal teas a more refreshing option.

Sometimes you have to persevere before you acquire a taste for something new but in the end it's worth it if you can find some caffeine free alternatives.

I am not saying cut out coffee and tea completely but, once again, try and find some balance.   Remember, it's the caffeine that can be dehydrating if taken to excess and this can work against your cleansing programme.

Also this diet is all about extending your choice, not limiting it, so finding a wider range of drinks will not only be more healthy for you but also more enjoyable.

Keep down the wheat

Cutting out or reducing wheat is difficult because it is in so many foods. Therefore the starting point has to be bread. If you can remove bread from your diet then this will be a great starting point.

That includes wholewheat bread. I understand that for some, removing bread will be difficult. However, there are some really tasty alternatives you can try. A visit to the local health shop is a good starting point although top supermarkets now have sections for wheat free bread and there is quite a good selection.

There are an array of breads and crispbreads that you can try. Yeast-free soda bread, bread from pumpernickel, rye bread, rice cakes, oat cakes, oat biscuits – there is a lot of choice.

If removing bread from your diet is too painful for you, try and limit it to just one slice per day. This will give you time to start introducing alternatives.

Bread aside, if you can remove things like biscuits, cakes and pastries completely then this is a very positive step. This will not only have an immediate, positive effect on your digestive system but also on other aspects of your health such as blood sugar balance and cholesterol!

Also, remember that wheat will be present in many breakfast cereals, some sausages, taramasalata to name a few, so always look at the label.

In an earlier chapter on wheat, I mentioned that many other of the grains such as oats, rye and barley have gluten. But these grains have benefits which outweigh the negatives so they can and should be eaten in moderation.

Oats for example do contain gluten but their soluble fibre content more than makes up for the mucus forming potential so they are worth having as part of your diet.

I will emphasise again that balance is the key to success. In my view it is better to vary your food. Most people can vary their evening meals but seem stuck with a fairly rigid regime for breakfast.

In conversations with people who call my office, a great many have just porridge every day. For the reasons mentioned before, my proposal is that breakfast, like other meals, should be varied and cereals like porridge should be consumed no more than three to four times per week, using other wheat free alternatives such as rye, barley, spelt and sprouted wheat on other days. Once again if you need some help with choices then visit your local health store who should have plenty of alternatives such as wheat free mueslis, rice cereals and millet flakes.

One of my favourite breakfasts these days is 'bubble and squeak.' I started this regime when I was looking to increase my intake of vegetables. I steam the veg the night before and then fry in olive oil in the morning. I do this perhaps twice per week and then have a grain type cereal such as porridge or muesli on other days.

If you get yourself a juicer, you can juice some organic apples and put this juice on your cereal instead of milk. It's a real treat.

Try cleansing vegetable soups

Making your own, healthy veggie soup is of course a great way to increase daily intake of cleansing foods. You can get some really good ideas from the Gerson therapy book. I have made reference to the Gerson therapy earlier. To reiterate – this is a therapy based on healing the body from serious disease by eliminating high mucus, highly acidic foods and replacing them with high cleansing, mucus free, alkaline foods i.e. lots of juices made from organic fruits, vegetables and salad foods.

Hippocrates soup is one of the most recommended soups. It is based on tomatoes, celery, garlic, potatoes, onions and leeks. It is a very powerful, cleansing soup.

The book contains other healthy options which you can get some ideas from.

Another way to increase your levels of cleansing food is to eat one good portion of fruit before every meal. Remember, fruit is cleansing, so by having that extra bit three times a day will go a long way to achieving your '10 a day' target.

By moving to a more fresh food diet, you will naturally get more fibre. If you want to accelerate the cleansing process then you can try soluble fibre products like psyllium husks and linseed or add pulses and beans to soup.

Make your own hummus with chickpeas, garlic and olive oil. You can increase your garlic consumption in general as this has a cleansing effect. Garlic is brilliant for helping to keep the fungus Candida under control and it is also effective in killing off parasites.

Remember, most convenience and readymade meals have wheat in them

For at least three evenings per week try and have fresh food like steamed fish and salad. Restrict convenience foods as much as possible. Perhaps on two days, have no fish or meat at all. This will of course not be difficult if you are a vegetarian!

Below is a list of standard supermarket foods which may contain wheat:

Bagels	Chocolate bars and sweets (candy)
Batter	Cheese biscuits (crackers) /Twiglets
Biscuits/Cookies	Couscous
Bread	Curry sauce/chilled/frozen curries
Bread sticks	Custard powder or sauce
Breakfast cereals	Doughnuts
Bulgar wheat	Dumplings
Cakes and Muffins	Durum wheat
Chapatti	Danish pastries
Crispbread	Egg noodles
Croissants	Fish in batter or breadcrumbs
Crumble mix	Fish pie
Cake and muffin mix	Frozen desserts
Cauliflower cheese	French bread and French toast

Gravy powder

Macaroni cheese and Lasagne

Mayonnaise (some)

Meat pies and puddings

Mexican dishes - enchiladas, wheat flour tortillas, nachos

Naan bread

Onion Bhajis (but wheat free in most Indian restaurants)

Pancakes or Crêpe

Pasta

Pasta sauce

Pastry

Pitta bread

Pizza crusts or bases

Pot noodles

Quiches

Sausages and sausage rolls

Seafood in breadcrumbs

Scotch eggs

Semolina

Soup

Spring rolls

Sauce mix

Steamed puddings

Scones and crumpets

Sliced processed ham, turkey and meats

Vegetables in batter (e.g. onion rings)

Vegetables in breadcrumbs (e.g. mushrooms)

Vegetarian frozen dishes

Vegetarian prepared foods

Waffles

Yorkshire puddings

Gluten free options

Let me emphasise again, for this diet to be successful, you do not have to give up all wheat but you have to give the pendulum a big swing away from it.

For those of you who want to go that step further and reduce wheat right down to an absolute minimum, below are some suggestions for gluten free options.

Rice – rice is of course one of the first options for most. You can get rice noodles and pasta these days and brown rice flour can be used very successfully for baking. Rice cakes are a useful snack option.

Corn – corn pasta is available in many different forms – penne, spaghetti, etc Cornflakes are a useful snack option (very occasionally) and cornflour can be used to thicken sauces.

Quinoa – is a good source of protein and you can use it like rice or use as flakes as an ingredient in muesli mixes. Quinoa flour and milk are now also available.

Buckwheat – this is available as flour, pasta and noodles. It can be used very successfully to make pancakes or wraps.

Millet – cook like porridge or add flakes to a muesli mix.

Potato - a useful starchy alternative to grains. Potato flour can be used to thicken sauces.

Chestnut - Chestnut flour can be used for baking or to thicken sauces.

Tapioca – from the cassava plant, this grain can be used to make pudding.

There are also a number of gluten free products on the market but gluten free doesn't always mean healthy. Look out for the additives and added sugars.

Dairy's next

As we have seen, dairy is perhaps the second main cause of mucus after wheat so it is important to get some dairy free options into your diet.

If you are concerned about leaving out dairy, then there are some things to consider.

Don't worry about your calcium intake if you cut dairy out. We've been lead to believe that without milk, our bones will crumble. The truth is that although dairy produce is high in calcium it is not a very good source of other minerals, particularly magnesium. Calcium and magnesium form a nutritional double-act, without one, the other simply cannot function. Relying on dairy produce for calcium is likely to lead to an imbalance in other minerals, certainly NOT the best idea for bone protection.

Calcium in combination with all the other minerals essential for bone health, can be found in many dietary sources, as shown below:

Sardines, almonds, watercress, parsley, sunflower seeds, quinoa, walnuts, salmon, eggs, brown rice, chicken and kelp. If in doubt, ask your local health store to recommend a good calcium/magnesium supplement combination.

So, if you can reduce dairy intake from milk, cream and cheese right down to a minimum, you will have gone a long way to cutting out a lot of mucus forming food.

Yoghurt is tolerated better and can be used occasionally. Soya yoghurts are an occasional alternative but, as mentioned before, soya itself can be very mucus forming so use in moderation.

General foods to avoid which might contain dairy

Milk and cream are the obvious ones. Also, cream is to be found in many soups so always read the label. There are good ranges of fresh soups in supermarkets and many of them are 'dairy free' so check this out.

Dairy is also found in most sauces, mousses, desserts, ice cream, sour cream, crème fraiche, dips, dressings and most chocolate.

If you like yoghurts then go for the bio versions. You can also alternate between soya and goat's varieties but whatever varieties you go for, try and avoid eating more than one fresh yoghurt every other day. There are benefits to these products but too many can add to the 'mucus' effect.

Try to avoid those sweetened, flavoured yoghurts which offer limited nutritional value.

With regards to milk, my favourite alternative is rice milk because it is so versatile although a little sweet. Oat milk is widely available as I'm sure you know but there are so many new varieties emerging in your health shop, they are worth a look. You can now get almond milk, quinoa milk and hazelnut milk.

If you can't leave cheese alone, hard is better than soft but try and keep this to an absolute minimum if you are serious about keeping your insides clean. Roquefort cheese and feta are some good alternatives but not every day. Say two or three days per week.

For a low fat spread use the brand Pure (free from wheat and dairy), or pumpkin seed butter, or non-hydrogenated spread such as Vitaquell. Also olive oil could be kept in the fridge and when it thickens you can use it as butter. Your local health shop will, I am sure, offer you some good choices – go and see for yourself. Some of the nut butters like Almond butter are just delicious in moderation.

Reduce meat – red meat in particular

For an on-going cleansing diet it is recommended that red meats and pork should, as far as possible, be eliminated from the diet.

Both meats have been linked to a higher risk of colon cancer so from this point alone you should consider cutting back if you are not already doing so.

You need to be particularly careful about mixed varieties of meat in sausages and pies.

Pies in particular, if consumed regularly have the potential to really clog your system.   You have the double whammy effect of the gluten in the pastry and the red meat.   This type of snack food is best avoided altogether.

So, the best types of meats are lean lamb and free range poultry. Of course fresh fish is the other main option.

Throughout the week, I would recommend that you have at least two days that are totally meat and fish free. This will give your system a really good chance to give itself a thorough cleanse on a regular basis.

If you are a vegetarian, remember not to substitute meat with too many carbohydrates. Concentrate on the proteins from seeds, pulses and nuts. There is a tendency amongst young vegetarians to eat lots more cheese and sticky buns which are two of the most mucus forming foods so - once again - variety is the key, making sure your sources of food are, as far as possible, free from wheat and dairy.

Reduce stodgy snacks

Well I think you have the idea now. Most of those lovely peanuts, crisps and pastries that you love to snack on are some of the major contributors to your system getting clogged – so you must make an effort and find some alternatives such as almonds, brazil nuts, hazelnuts, sunflower seeds and pumpkin seeds.

Just one trip to your health shop will also reveal a whole host of snacks based on rice and oats that will be so much healthier for you.

Most nuts are fine and a great source of protein. There is no need to go hungry. Try and make sure you always have a small bag of almonds around so you can snack on them when peckish – they are also great to keep your blood sugars stable as I have said earlier.

I can't emphasise enough that this change in diet has nothing to do with restricting choice. In fact, if I do my job properly - and you do yours - you will be eating a much wider selection of foods.

Some of the alternative choices you find might be more expensive – but how do you evaluate your health?

Also, if you add up how much you spend on some of those stodgy snacks and pastries, you might be surprised. You might find that by getting a weekly delivery of organic vegetables and fruit to your home your food bill will go down.

I certainly spend less on buying foods 'on the go' since I arranged to get regular supplies of organic fruit and veg delivered to my door. Foods 'on the go' can be expensive. My baguette at lunch time costs £1.50. I now save between £20.00 and £30.00 pounds per month by taking a mixture of my own cooked vegetables or vegetable soup to work. So, some sensible healthy choices can save you money.

Your desire for sweet, sugary foods will evaporate.

Once you have given up those stodgy cakes and pastries and enjoyed the invigorating boost that you get from a 'home made' organic juice, you will thank me. You will begin to really taste the difference between fresh, live food and that which is nutritionally dead and artificially sweet.

Most of us have a sweet tooth to some degree and I am no exception but you can go a long way to satisfying this with honey, maple syrup and choices like blackstrap molasses.

One sweetener, xylitol, is better than most. It has quite a unique quality for a bulk sweetener in that it has a low glycaemic index. This means that it does not cause major blood sugar fluctuations like most sugars or sweeteners. You can buy it in bulk from health shops.

Don't eat five portions of fruit and vegetables a day, make it ten!

As you will have gathered, I am recommending that fruit, vegetables and salad should start to make up a large percentage of your diet. In the media it's all about five portions a day but on your on-going cleansing diet, you should be aiming for at least 10 portions a day and more if you include salad foods.

Vegetables that are particularly good from a 'cleansing' point of view are cabbage, onion, artichokes and chicory because they all contain an ingredient called inulin, a prebiotic, which has a 'probiotic' effect once in your large bowel. This means it helps you to produce your own 'friendly' bacteria. Carrots should also play a major part in your diet.

Probiotic activity is another weapon in the armoury to countering any mucus that is forming in the stool.

I will explain more about prebiotics in Chapter 10.

Remember to have lots of vegetables available at all times. This means they are to hand when you need a snack so you can choose these rather than biscuits or wheat crispbreads.

Instead of wheat biscuits try raw carrots, broccoli, celery, cucumber and peppers with dips like hummus and guacamole.

If you don't want to give up the crispbreads, there are oat based biscuits which you can use. These are of course wheat free but they also have a low glycaemic index so they are better for your blood sugar levels as well.

Varying your intake of vegetables is important. Other good choices are brussel sprouts, different types of cabbage, cauliflower, asparagus, artichokes, sweet potatoes, carrots, swede, leeks and onions.

It's amazing how tasty you can make vegetable soup just by getting a really good mix of vegetables together. Adding spices like turmeric, ginger and cayenne pepper will also add extra health benefits.

Occasionally, adding beans to the mix is a good idea. A portion of beans such as kidney beans or lentils can be counted as one of your vegetable portions. Beans are a great source of protein - as they have good cleansing properties and are nutrient rich.

On the fruit side of things, once again, variety is the key. Oranges, pineapples, apples, berry fruits, papaya, melon, fresh or dried figs, prunes, pears, strawberries, kiwi fruit, melon and raisins are all good choices. Bananas are considered to be slightly mucus forming so maybe no more than three per week. They are however really good in smoothies.

Grapes and citrus fruits are some of the greatest mucus-cleansers. They help the body to remove toxins and supply vital nutrients in the correct balance for rejuvenation and healing.

Without the natural, sponge-like properties of fruit and vegetables, intestinal diseases will continue to abound, especially amongst the elderly. Ironically as people get older and depend more on other people, they probably are inclined to eat more convenience foods and less fresh fruit and vegetables. Constipation in the elderly is a major problem for those running care homes. Often the 'quick fix' is used which is not pleasant for anyone involved!

By making fresh fruit and vegetables – preferably organic - the major part of your diet, you will be empowering your body to remove mucus from the intestines and cleanse your whole elimination system – including the lymph glands.

Remember the salad options

For those of you who are calorie conscious, you could use salads to help you reach your goal of ten fruit and vegetables per day.

Salads are usually served at the beginning of a meal, but a salad can also make a healthy, low-calorie meal all by itself. The key to keeping salads interesting is to change the ingredients each time you make one. Don't just think of the simple garden salad, but imagine adding fruits, nuts and occasionally lean meats, to your salad to make a great low-calorie, highly nutritious meal.

Most salads start with a pile of greens. Since greens are low in calories and are a good source of fibre, this is a great way to add volume to your meal without adding a lot of calories. There are different varieties of lettuce, such as iceberg, leaf, spinach, escarole, romaine, or butter. The darker lettuces offer more vitamins than pale iceberg, for example. Spinach has iron, and all varieties are low in calories. One cup of shredded lettuce has about 5 to 10 calories.

Almost any raw vegetable can be cut up and added to a salad. Green beans, snap peas, carrots, radishes, broccoli, cauliflower, zucchini, asparagus, artichokes, avocados, tomatoes, and cucumbers are all great suggestions. As you are going to need at least ten servings of fruits and vegetables per day, eating a salad is a good way to meet those needs. Brightly coloured vegetables have bioflavonoids, and the dark green vegetables are lowest in calories - about 20 calories per half cup serving.

On the fruit side, blueberries, raspberries, blackberries, apple slices and raisins add vitamins and antioxidants. The delicious burst of flavour and sweetness they add can also help you cut back on, or eliminate, high-calorie salad dressings. A half cup of apple slices has 30 calories, and a half cup of berries has about 40 calories.

Healthy protein sources

To make a meal of a salad, you may wish to add some healthy protein sources like chopped or sliced hard-boiled eggs, tuna, or lean chicken breast.

Sprinkle a few nuts like walnuts, pecans, almonds or pine nuts for a nice crunch. Just a few nuts will do, about one-eighth cup of nuts adds about 90 calories. Walnuts are a great source of omega-3 essential fatty acids, and all of the nuts add protein and heart-healthy polyunsaturated fatty acids.

For salad dressing, the best option is to use olive oil or organic flax seed oil as your dressing. However, a salad with a variety of fruits and vegetables really doesn't need any dressing; some freshly squeezed lemon or lime juice will likely be enough to suit your taste.

Here is a great example of a delicious, healthy salad for you to try:
- two cups of green leaf lettuce
- one-fourth cup raw green beans
- one-fourth cup snap peas
- one-fourth cup chopped tomato
- one-fourth cup sliced carrots
- one-fourth cup apple slices
- one-fourth cup blueberries
- one-fourth cup chopped chicken breast or one ounce of shredded mozzarella cheese
- one boiled egg
- one-eighth cup walnut pieces
- lemon and lime wedges

This salad has lots of vitamins, antioxidants, phytochemicals and fibre and comes in at just under 400 calories.

Salads can be changed and adapted to any diet. If you are watching your calories choose the lowest calorie ingredients. Keep lots of salad fruits and vegetables on hand, and you will find it easy to create salads several times per week. Change the ingredients to create completely different flavours, and you will never get bored with healthy salad meals.

Invest in a juicer if you have problems with digestion

If you have had a serious illness or are on any long term medication from your doctor and feel that you are not absorbing nutrients effectively from your food, then you should definitely consider investing in a juicer (you may have heard me mention this a few times in this book)!

You can juice most vegetables and fruits. The advantage of pure juices is that they do not require normal digestion. Even an impaired digestive system will quickly absorb the juice and its nutrients. Also, they taste absolutely wonderful and a juice of apples, carrots, celery and cucumber is a really refreshing way to start the day. Even most greens taste fine when juiced with apples. Any good juice book will give you all the alternatives you will need.

By increasing the vegetable and fruit content of your diet you will not only be moving towards a cleaner digestive tract, you will also be moving towards a cleaner, healthier body – one which is less prone to disease.

Make the changes gradually

If your diet has been very much a red meat eater's diet or one which included pastries and crisps, then you will probably get quite depressed reading all this if you are really keen to change your diet as there will be so many changes to make.

I am not advocating that you make these changes overnight. If you can introduce things gradually over a few months so that the emphasis of your diet is changing toward a more cleansing diet then this is probably the best way if you are going to stick to it. This will give time for your tastes to adapt. There are lots of choices once you know where to get them and you will probably find yourself eating a more varied diet once you get organised.

In Chapter 10, I outline some natural ingredients that can accelerate the cleansing process whilst you are trying to sort out your new regime.

There is never any need to go hungry – once you start experimenting you will find plenty of alternatives to eat and snack on.

Below, I am summarising a few pointers for you.

Foods to eat regularly:

- Pineapple and papaya, for the digestive system. They are ideal as a starter for all meals.
- Garlic, to cleanse the digestive tract.
- Black cherries, blueberries, cranberries and black grapes, to heal the digestive tract (these also contain large amounts of antioxidant nutrients).
- Cabbage, broccoli, carrots, asparagus, which provide multiple benefits including soluble fibre and antioxidant nutrients. They are also very good for the digestive system.
- Sprouted seeds, as a source of enzymes and good quality/low fat protein.
- Quinoa, for a virtually fat-free source of protein.
- Green leafy vegetables and nuts (not peanuts), for calcium and magnesium.

Foods to eat occasionally:

- Live (bio) yoghurt to provide friendly bacterial for the digestive tract. Yoghurt is also a good source of protein.
- Soya products such as tofu, soya yoghurts, soya milk etc.,
- Rice and oat milk.

Some do's:

- Drink 2.0 litres of pure still water each day, but not during main meals.
- Eat breakfast before work, don't leave it till mid-morning.
- Snack on a handful of mixed seeds, nuts and raisins each day. Also snack on fresh fruit and vegetables (celery, carrots, cucumber, tomatoes etc).
- Keep wheat-free emergency snacks like hummus and guacomole with oat biscuits.

- Drink herb tea when you are thirsty, stressed or need warming up.
- Eat fruit before each meal.

Do: Eat salads, soups, baked potatoes or dairy free dips with raw vegetables for lunch and not sandwiches.

Do: Go for a brisk walk after lunch, but relax and unwind after dinner.

Do: Eat fish two to three times a week

Some don'ts

- Drink tea or coffee more than three times per day.
- Drink fizzy or cola type drinks.
- Snack on breads, biscuits, cookies, doughnuts, pastries and chocolate.
- Add salt to your food or eat salty foods (processed or junk foods or chips/crisps).
- Eat fresh fruit until 2 hours after a meat course.
- Snack within 20 minutes of a main meal.
- Eat mayonnaise.
- Bolt your food. Chew it and enjoy it!
- Eat meat more than three times a week.

Well, lots of food for thought, but the question is – is your new diet going to be balanced? Does it provide you with a good balance of carbohydrates, protein and fats?

Let's see.

CHAPTER 10

Is Your New Diet Balanced?

So, by changing your diet to one that has a far higher percentage of vegetables and fruit, are you going to get a balanced diet? Are you getting a good balance of carbohydrates, protein, fat and fibre? Let's take a look at your carbohydrates first.

Complex carbohydrates – you'll get plenty

Firstly, your new diet will give you lots and lots of energy because you will be getting lots of complex carbohydrates from it. You will get this from your extra portions of fruit and vegetables and of course those bean mixes you are putting into your vegetable soup.

Your oat and millet cereals will also provide you with a good supply of complex carbohydrates and having rice, baked potatoes and lentils on an occasional basis will also give you lots of complex carbohydrates as well.

Also, remember to have that extra bit of fruit before your cereal in the morning.

Having a good intake of complex carbohydrates is better for your blood sugar and also your general health than the simple sugars you get in sweets and many cereals.

Complex carbohydrates enter your blood stream more slowly and over a longer period of time. The result is that your blood sugar does not fluctuate so widely and this makes it more stable. This is why avoiding the typical wheat puddings, such as chocolate sponge which contains lots of white flour, is not only good from a mucus point of view it is also good for blood sugar.

Too much refined sugar – like you get in stodgy puddings and in some breads - can cause large fluctuations in blood sugar and over a long period of time can have health implications. In fact the high refined sugar intake in the West these days, which you often get in fast food restaurants, is believed to be one of the causes of the massive increase in the number of cases of Type 2 Diabetes.

So, no problem on the complex carbohydrates with your new diet.

Your new diet will give you the US target of 50g of fibre per day.

No problem with fibre either. I have covered the fibre aspect of your diet in other chapters but it suffices to say that if you are consuming between eight and ten pieces of fruit and vegetables daily and all those nuts, beans and salad foods, you should be getting loads of natural soluble fibre. This will be enhanced by the better choice of cereals you will be choosing.

Your new diet should be helping you achieve over 50g of fibre per day - more than twice what the average person in the UK consumes.

What about your protein?

Then there's protein. You cannot live without protein - you need it to survive. The fact is that most of us probably eat too much protein – particularly red meat protein and when we do this, it can be one of the major contributors to a mucus forming diet.

If you eat meat most days you may be concerned that I am recommending that you only eat meat on two to three days per week. Are you getting sufficient protein if you do this?

The fact is that you will be getting more than sufficient quality protein from the eggs (three times per week) fish (three times per week) along with the extra beans and pulses.

On the days that you do eat meat, try and go for lean chicken, turkey, venison and lamb. These will be better for you than beef and pork from a mucus point of view.

My recommendation would be, throughout the week, you try and eat meat no more than two to three times concentrating more on fish, beans and eggs. Eggs are arguably the most perfect protein you can eat but here again, three per week should be sufficient. So the secret is to spread these sources of protein throughout the week and if you do this sensibly, then you will be getting all the healthy protein your body needs.

Also, if you are vegetarian, you can add Quinoa, an excellent source of protein, to your porridge or other cereal in the mornings. Mixing lentils with rice gives you the complete complex carbohydrate and protein mix.

And as my vegetarian friends keep pointing out – vegetables and plants also contain protein!   The largest mammal on this planet –the elephant – is vegetarian, so they must be getting plenty of protein from somewhere!

But what about your fat intake?

Certain types of fat will be very important to your new diet

Although my dietary recommendations will mean that you will be cutting out certain types of fats, there are others that will be important to your cleansing diet and also important to your health.

Fat really is crucial in your diet - it's needed for helping you absorb essential vitamins A, D, E and K; and for maintaining healthy skin and body functions, including immunity and brain development. It's also a major source of energy, as well as keeping you warm and protecting your organs.

Fat also makes food appetising.

When it comes to your new cleansing diet it is very important to understand which fats are good and those that are bad.

Too much focus in recent years has been on reducing fat particularly with so many low-fat meals.   If your body doesn't get enough of the right fats you will not be healthy and research has shown you are more likely to be depressed.

The last thing you want to do is clog yourself up with bad fat but also, at the same time, I don't want you to make yourself ill by not taking in enough of the good fats.

I want to spend a bit more time on this subject as it is so important to get it right.

The bad fats

Saturated Fat

All fats are made up of carbon, hydrogen and oxygen, buts it's the proportions of these that have a different effect on the body. Saturated fats are so called because they're saturated with hydrogen atoms. This kind of fat is usually hard at room temperature - think lard.

Saturated fat is found in animal foods such as meat and dairy - particularly cheese, butter, cream and full fat milk - but also some oils, including coconut oil (used in many shop-bought baked products).

The reason that lots of saturated fat is bad for you is that excessive consumption can increase mucus in your system and also increase levels of bad cholesterol in the blood, which increases the risk of coronary heart disease. A government report from January 2008 concluded that cutting our intake of saturated fat could save 3500 lives in Britain a year.

Not everyone agrees that this link has been adequately proven. The general consensus though is that we should cut down. The average guideline daily amount (GDA) for men is 30g, and for women 20g, but the Food Standards Agency say we're eating 20% too much on average.

And when you consider a fried breakfast with buttered toast and a cappuccino contains 33.7g, it's not hard to notch up those fat grams.

So, you need to cut down on cakes, biscuits and other baked products, trim excess fat off meat and avoid too much cream and fatty cheese.

Saturated fat and your new cleansing diet

Well, the great thing is that by following your cleansing diet you will automatically be removing most of the 'bad' fats – those that clog up your arteries and your digestive tract. The worst offenders – red meat, cheese, milk etc will automatically be omitted or at least reduced drastically from your diet. So this is a good start.

There is some saturated fat in eggs but, as I have said before, the plus side of eggs by far outweighs the negatives. As I keep saying, perhaps no more than three per week would be about right.

The next bad fat is known commonly as 'trans fat.'

Trans Fat

Trans fat is created when vegetable (unsaturated) oil is partially hydrogenated, giving it a higher melting point and making it more solid. These fats are used in some foods to give them a longer shelf life.

They are very unstable but they are however very adaptable and this is one reason why they are used extensively in pastries and processed foods – the two food categories that I am recommending you give a wide berth to.

Trans fat is found in some processed foods such as biscuits and cakes, cheese, meat pies and pastries.

Margarines all used to contain trans fats but most manufacturers have reformulated in recent years because of the bad publicity surrounding them and their harmful effects. They are considered to be a major cause of hardening of the arteries and heart disease.

Some meat products and dairy foods also contain trans fats

These fats block your arteries and block the good effects of the good fats (omega 3).

Therefore it is wise to avoid any low fat spreads or margarine if hydrogenated fat is mentioned on the ingredients.

Although they are unsaturated in terms of chemical make-up, these fats don't have any health benefits.

Once again, your new diet, if followed to a reasonable level, will steer you away from pies, pastries and processed foods so once again you will be avoiding this harmful fat.

The good news is that the food industry has reduced its use of trans fats in recent years and the average person in the UK eats below the recommended level. But it's still worth checking food labels on processed foods and cutting out trans or partially hydrogenated fats.

We have now looked at the two main bad fats- now let's look at the good guys.

The Good Fats

Polyunsaturated Fat

Poly fats are known as essential fats, quite simple because they're vital for our health. Our bodies can't produce them, so we need to get them from our diet. There are two types: omega-3 and omega-6

Omega-6 is found in vegetable oils including sunflower, safflower and corn oils, nuts and seeds, meat and chicken;

Omega-3 is in flaxseed and raspeseed oil, nuts, green vegetables and oily fish such as sardines, mackerel, salmon and fresh tuna.

Polyunsaturated fat helps reduce the 'bad' (LDL) cholesterol in your blood, helping to protect against heart disease. Omega-3 helps our brains and eyes to function well.

Omega-6 helps with growth, immunity and healthy skin, as well as our reproductive system.

Most of us eat enough omega-6-rich foods, but lack omega-3. This is mainly because many people don't eat enough oily fish although many believe you can get good quality omega-3 from flax seed oil. Current advice is to eat three portions of fish a week, one of which should be oily.

If you don't like fish, consider taking a supplement. For vegetarians, flaxseed oil is the best option.

Polyunsaturated fat and your new diet

Throughout this book I am trying to steer you to consume fish for your protein rather than meat and this will help your Omega-3 intake.

Omega-3 is important because it is not only healthy but helps you feel good as well. There is growing evidence that low levels of Omega-3 can have a detrimental effect on your brain activity and this can lead to depression. For those of you who are concerned about eating too much fish because of the potential pollutants, you can now purchase purified fish oil – in the form of E-EPA which will provide you with the benefits of Omega-3 without the potential downsides of pollution in fish.

Fortunately if you follow the cleansing diet I am recommending, you will be getting plenty of Omega-3 fatty acids from your fish, nuts and seeds intake. However, as this fat is so important to your health I would recommend topping up with organic flax seed oil or a purified fish oil like E-EPA which I have mentioned above.

By replacing saturated fats with unsaturated fats you can improve your heart health as well as your bowel health. Remember, essential fatty acids are good for your brain, your joints, your metabolism and for a stable blood sugar.

Recent research has shown that regular intake of Omega-3 fatty acids reduces the incidence of colon cancer.

If you are a vegetarian then you will have to work hard to get your essential fats from seeds, nuts and flax seed oil.

Monounsaturated fat

This is a type of unsaturated fat, and is typically liquid at room temperature. The most common mono fat in our diets is oleic acid, otherwise known as Omega-9.

Sources of Omega-9 are olives and olive oil, nuts, avocados, many vegetable oil spreads and rapeseed oil.

The Mediterranean diet is high in mono fats and this has been linked to low blood pressure and lower incidences of heart disease. Experts say mono fat helps reduce levels of unhealthy cholesterol. These fats are associated with a reduced risk of colon cancer and heart disease.

Putting generous helpings of olive oil on your salads and other foods can be good for your health. It is also safe for frying if you use small amounts. It is a good all-round cooking oil but has a low smoke point so it can't be used for deep frying. 'Extra Virgin' olive oil means that the oil has come from first the pressing of the fruit and is the most flavoursome.

If you put it in the fridge it will solidify and some people use this as an alternative to butter.

Another benefit of olive oil for those of you trying to lose a few pounds – according to new research – is that it can help to keep you slim. This is according to a study reported in the journal 'Cell Metabolism.' It's thought that a fatty acid found in the oil, called oleic acid, stimulates the production of a chemical that sends messages to the brain saying you are full. Oleic acid is also found in grapeseed oil and avocados. Scientists hope this discovery could help overweight people while the study authors don't recommend glugging neat olive oil to keep hunger pangs at bay, but switching to olive oil as your main cooking oil will be beneficial for you health and weight.

Your new diet and monounsaturated fat

A Mediterranean diet, overall, is far more balanced than other European cuisine from a cleansing point of view. Lots of fresh salads lend themselves to some type of dressing and olive oil should figure prominently here rather than the more creamy alternatives such as thousand island and mayonnaise which are clogging and mucus forming.

The Mediterranean diet is high in mono fats and these, as I have mentioned earlier, have been linked to low blood pressure and lower incidences of heart and bowel disease.

Monounsaturated fat may also be associated with a reduced risk of developing certain cancers.

Healthy Oils

So, oils can play an important part in your new diet and olive oil and flaxseed oil should figure prominently. One other oil – Hemp seed oil – is also a healthy option and should also be considered. It contains Omega-3, 6 and 9 essential fatty acids so it's another oil that could be particularly useful if you want some variety.

I know that many of you when trying to reduce dairy, find it difficult to reduce butter particularly when using it on baked potatoes and the like. However, you should try organic flax oil in situations like this. It has a nutty taste and really brings out the taste of a baked potato. It is a versatile oil and the more you use it the more uses you will find for it.

How your PH balance is helped by your new cleansing diet

Well, I have talked a lot about mucus forming foods and how they can clog not only your bowels but also your whole body.

I am now going to talk about your 'PH' balance.

If you are not into food science then you probably haven't heard this term since your chemistry days at school.

Many nutritionists and naturopaths are now using the PH balance of the intercellular liquid in your body as a measure of your health.

A lot of the interest in PH balance has been by the American microbiologist, Robert Young, who recently produced a book entitled The PH Miracle.

What this book is saying is that if your body's tissues become over 'acidic' then this means in simple terms that you will be more prone to disease.

This over-acidification can be corrected by adopting a PH balancing diet.

The great thing about all this is that your new 'cleansing' diet falls totally into line with a PH balancing diet.

Let me explain in a little more detail.

There is a growing belief that the main contributor to many of today's diseases such as arthritis, fatigue, heart disease and possibly cancer, is an over-acidification in the PH of the body's tissues.

What is PH exactly?

This is the measure of how acidic or alkaline something is. You can measure it on a scale of 0-14. A PH of 7 is neutral. A PH lower than 7 is acidic and a PH above 7 is alkaline.

What we are talking about here is the acid-alkaline balance of the fluids within and surrounding the cells within your body. This could be, according to Robert Young, the key to health.

We are not talking about the acid in your stomach for example where the acid levels are of course a lot higher. Also, the environment within a healthy bowel is quite acid.

But over half of the fluid in your body is intracellular fluid and this is slightly alkaline at around 7.

If your diet is too acid forming then your body has the ability to neutralise the excess to keep the PH balance alkaline.

If however over many years the amount of acid forming foods exceeds the body's ability to neutralise and remove it, the body will resort to other measures to maintain an alkaline PH. This might include dumping acid in certain body tissues (fat is an easy option) causing cellulite and drawing on minerals such as magnesium, potassium and calcium from other parts of the body.

So, the type of diet that could over time put a strain on your body by making it too acidic is very similar to the mucus forming diet I have been mentioning throughout this book.

I refer to the diet of our prehistoric ancestors in chapter ten. Genetically our bodies are still geared up for our predominantly plant based hunter-gatherer diet that relied on root vegetables, bulbs and berries and meat only occasionally.

The move to a grain based diet – which is more acid forming - started around 10,000 years ago.

Eating acid forming foods is not an issue for your health provided the acid part of your diet does not dominate.

Unfortunately in the last hundred years or so, the intake of grains and animal products has snow-balled and the consumption of our plant based products has fallen.

When I make reference to acid forming foods, people often make reference to fruit like oranges and grapefruit as these are foods that you normally associate with as being 'high acid content.'

However, the acidity in your cells relates more to how food is handled by your body. As a general comment, fruit (yes, even grapefruit) has an alkalising effect in the body. On the other hand grains, meat, seafood and eggs are acid forming.

Let's have a look to see in which category the most common foods fall.

Acid-forming foods:

All meat products, eggs, cheese, milk, nuts, some seeds, lentils, peas, tofu, chick peas (only slight) and grains (oat flakes, buckwheat whole grain, rye, spelt, wheat bran, millet, rice and corn).

Out of these, most of the grain products (with the exception of wheat and bran), spelt, eggs, nuts (not peanuts or cashews), lentils and chick peas can be part of your new cleansing diet but, once again, not the major part.

Alkaline-forming foods:

All vegetables, beans (especially white, pinto, lima, mung and kidney), fruits (figs, plums, prunes, raisins and avocados are the most alkaline-forming), grains (buckwheat flour and quinoa), green beans, garlic, basil, chives, parsley, ginger, black pepper, apple cider vinegar and honey.

There are also alkalising supplements you can take such as: Magnesium, potassium and calcium, Chlorella, spirulina and other greens.

Your new diet and your PH balance

You guessed it. With only one or two exceptions, those foods which tend to be more mucus forming also have an acidifying effect on your body.

In the Western world it is estimated that our diets are around 70-75% acid forming and 25-30% alkalising.

For good health, this ratio needs to be reversed so that your diet is only 25-30% acid forming and 75-80% alkalising.

We are now reverting back to this balance thing again. There are many mucus and acid forming foods such as eggs and oats that are perfectly healthy foods and can and should be an important part of your diet.

However, they should not be the major part.

This is where my recommendation of consuming at least 10 portions of fruits and vegetables per day on your cleansing diet comes in. You will need to get to these levels in order to get to the point when 70-75% of your diet is made up of cleansing, alkalising foods.

So my recommendations for your mucus free diet are spot-on to help you achieve the perfect PH balance.

Your new diet scores well in all five categories

The great thing about your new diet is that not only is it going to make you healthier, you should also feel the benefits in a very short period of time.

It will also give you a perfectly healthy, balanced diet.

But how long will it take to improve your bowel transit time? The truth of the matter is that everyone is different and so responses will be varied.

A system that has been clogged up over many years may take longer to clear so patience may be required. Cleansing your system naturally is not going to work overnight like a drug, particularly if you have been taking laxatives for a period of time. Laxatives can knock your natural peristalsis action and your natural rhythm. The secret about coming off laxatives is to wean yourself off them slowly.

In situations like this, or if you have a really sluggish system that only responds every few days, you may need some help in the form of some natural food supplements whilst you take time to move over to, and get used to, your new diet.

I am going to recommend just five different groups of nutrients which, when combined together, will overcome even the most stubborn constipation. They will also work to improve your bowel health over a period of time.

As all five are from natural sources they can be taken alongside your new diet, as required.

CHAPTER 11

Some natural ingredients that can help cleanse your system

By the end of this book, I am hoping that you will have sufficient information to counteract any mucus forming influence you have in your system and that you will be able to adjust your diet to prevent a toxic build up from taking place in the future.

I appreciate that this might take a while and, as I keep saying, it is best if you can plan the changes over a period of time.

There are however, certain natural ingredients that you can take that can accelerate the process of cleansing your system and make it easier to swing the pendulum in your favour.

Some ten years ago I discovered three natural ingredients which, when taken together, were instrumental in helping me overcome my debilitating Irritable Bowel Syndrome which had plagued me for more than three years. It is no coincidence that these three ingredients are also extremely effective in reducing the impact of mucus development and any subsequent putrefaction.

Because of this I am recommending to you these three ingredients, plus two more, which will help you. They will help you to break down your food and digest it more efficiently, prevent putrefaction and any mucus build up in your digestive tract and also help you pass stools more easily without any artificial stimulation.

Recommendation 1:

Overcome bloating and get more out of the food you eat with a helping hand from a digestive enzyme complex.

The first natural supplement I am going to recommend is a digestive enzyme complex. The reason for this is that many of us, particularly those of us over 50, may not be producing enzymes at sufficient levels to break down our foods and absorb nutrients as efficiently as we would like. Also, as I mentioned in Chapter 3, enzymes required to digest certain foods are now sadly lacking in much of our fresh food.

So helping to correct these deficiencies can be a very important first step for your new digestive and bowel cleansing programme.

All health food shops stock a wide array of digestive enzyme complexes. I am sure that your local store will be only too happy to give you advice on this subject.

Traditional plant remedies can be helpful too. The papaya leaf is known to help protein digestion and soothe dyspepsia and gastritis. Ginger has also been found to ease pain, reduce inflammation and stimulate gastric secretions, and fenugreek seed has been traditionally used to ease stomach pains. Incidentally, the seeds of fenugreek have also been shown to stimulate enzyme secretion.

But if all this is too much hassle, a good digestive enzyme complex will do the job for you.

Recommendation 2:

Probiotics – our 'pro-life' friendly guys who can help you to smell nice

Next I am going to recommend our friendly probiotic bacteria which I suspect that you know all about. In fact there are over 500 different types but there are five that are known to have significant importance. These are Lactobacillus acidophilus, Lactobacillus rhamnosus, Lactobacillus plantarum, Lactobacillus bulgaricus and Bifidobacterium bifidum.

The weight of bacteria in your colon is estimated to be around 2lbs, which is pretty significant.

The crucial thing about any balance is to try and make sure that the good things exceed the bad. So it's your job to try and make sure that the largest percentage of your bacteria is made up of the good guys.

In a healthy gut the good bacteria will outnumber the bad bacteria and keep them in check.

Good bacteria helps peristalsis which means if they are in short supply, the digestive process slows down creating an environment which favours putrefaction and mucus production.

Low levels of good bacteria can in fact be the starting point of a toxic colon and can make you smell!

Symptoms of a bad bacterial overgrowth

Bad body odour, smelly feet in particular, excessive gas, bloating and awful smelling stools. These symptoms are a real sign of putrefaction and excessive levels of bad bacteria, as I have mentioned before.

By following the guidelines in this book and eating a diet that is less mucus forming, you're a step towards keeping the balance of good and bad bacteria in your favour.

Topping up with a probiotic supplement is something I would recommend for anyone over 50. According to recent research, our levels of good bacteria start to deplete after this age.

If you have been constipated for some time or have had consistent diarrhoea then you are likely to have an imbalance of bacteria in your gut. This means a greater risk of disease, infection and digestive disruption. Good bacteria transform lots of nasty substances, including putrefactive waste, into harmless wastes ready for discharge from the body.

There is now strong evidence that good bacteria can strengthen the immune system and improve the digestion of lactose (milk sugar). Anything that can help to digest milk will help in the overall process of reducing mucus. But probiotics have benefits in so many ways; I believe that everyone should be taking them, particularly sufferers of constipation or diarrhoea!

Keeping the good bacteria high with good probiotic supplements should, in my opinion, be a priority for everyone who suffers from constipation. Even if you don't want to take them every day, then certainly load up on them if you are going abroad where the water is a bit 'iffy'.

A few years ago I went with a large family group to Egypt for a wedding. If you've never been there before, then Egypt is notorious for getting tummy upsets which can ruin an otherwise absolutely wonderful experience!

As you might expect, those who topped up with supplements of good bacteria prior to departure fared far better than those who didn't, as far as tummy upsets were concerned. In fact, much much better!

Probiotics are not new. The discovery that certain types of bacteria could contribute to the health of the intestines and help ward off disease was first made way back in 1908 by the Russian scientist, Elis Metchnikoff. He was the first to use the term dysbiosis to indicate an imbalance of gut bacteria. Since then more than ten thousand papers have been published demonstrating the benefits of friendly flora.

What causes us to be depleted of this wonderful bacteria?

Antibiotics - it is now well reported that antibiotics can be harmful to the health of your bowels. This is because they knock out the good guys as well as the bad. If you are prescribed antibiotics then remember to top up with good bacteria to help prevent depletion. But don't take the probiotics and antibiotics together. Leave a gap of around six hours.

In normal circumstances, healthy bacteria can be easily replenished with a good diet but if you must have regular prescriptions then you should seriously consider a proper supplementation programme. Otherwise the short and long term health of your bowels could be compromised.

Mucus build-up becomes far more likely when bad bacteria exceeds the good.

Many other medicines affect bowel function and so probiotic supplementation should be the first thing to consider when transit time grinds to a halt.

As I say continually throughout this book, no one thing is going to overcome your constipation once and for all. It is usually a combination of things that will work. Some changes can be challenging and others more simple.

One of the easiest things you can do is to take probiotic supplements and once again I recommend that everyone do this. In my experience a good probiotic supplement programme can play a significant role in overcoming toxic constipation.

The reason for this is that the friendly bacteria and the bad bacteria (putrefactive bacteria) in the intestinal tract contradict and counteract each other in various ways. Friendly bacteria live on carbohydrates, whereas putrefactive bacteria live on protein.

Putrefactive bacteria do not grow well in the acid medium produced by friendly bacteria. However, the metabolism of protein by the putrefactive bacteria produces ammonia, which neutralises the acidity produced by the friendly bacteria.

If your diet is too high with protein like red meat, then it may take a vigorous growth of friendly bacteria in the intestinal tract to finally take control over the bad, putrefactive bacteria. Good quality protein is of course crucial but if the proportion of the wrong type of protein such as red meat gets too high, then the potential for the build up of putrefactive bacteria grows.

This is why the very high meat protein diets would be a disaster for your bowels and your health in the long term.

Two tips:

1. Take probiotic supplements, of course. Yoghurts that contain live culture are a good move but they contain very low levels.

Try and avoid flavoured yoghurts as they have so many 'undesirables' added. Taking probiotic supplements that contain a number of different strains appears to have the best effects.

2. For your meat protein, go organic when you can to avoid the antibiotics that are added to certain animal feeds. But, if you follow your new cleansing diet, this should not be a problem as you will not be eating much meat anyway!

So, probiotics are vital in the fight to overcoming constipation but there are several studies that now show that probiotics work better alongside other natural ingredients.

Fibre is particularly important for creating the right type of moist environment for healthy bacteria to proliferate and there is one type of fibre in particular that is better than all others in achieving this – psyllium husks.

We are all told to eat more fibre and throughout this book I have emphasised the fact that most people fall well below the US recommended daily levels of more than 35g per day.

I read recently that we, in the UK, tend to eat on average less that 15g per day. This is a significant difference and it just goes to show that if our fibre levels are that low, they are playing an insignificant role in our diet in general.

Hopefully, by now, you are starting to consider introducing plenty of fresh food with particular emphasis on cleansing fruits and vegetables. This will automatically mean more fibre.

This transition to a more cleansing diet might take some time. In my case, my dietary habits have changed gradually over the last 10 years and I know that my diet today is much healthier than before.

However, like most people I have busy schedules and it is not possible to eat right all the time, especially when travelling.

I probably need more fibre than most. I put this down to the Irritable Bowel Syndrome problems I had some years ago but even before that, I tended to be more on the sluggish side. However, just by supplementing my diet with two types of healthy fibres, I can easily reach the daily recommendations and all the benefits that go with them.

Recommendation 3:
Psyllium – the Rolls Royce of fibre

The third natural ingredient I am going to recommend is psyllium husk.

This is the first fibre that I myself rely on when I feel my fibre intake needs a top-up. If you have read anything that I have written before then you will know that I always refer to this plant as the 'Rolls Royce' of fibre simply because, in my view, it really is the best.

The reason for this is that it is an extremely gentle fibre. I refer to it as a 'chamois leather' rather than the 'brillo effect' you can get with bran fibre. It absorbs more water than any other fibre. In fact it absorbs a staggering 25 times its own weight in water.

Remember that the emphasis these days is on soluble fibre because of the extra health benefits it brings. The great thing about psyllium is that it is good for both constipation and diarrhoea. Most people find this difficult to understand.

In the case of constipation waste matter hangs around far too long in the large bowel. This means it gets too dry and becomes hard and difficult to pass.

Just by taking psyllium husk, waste that arrives in the large colon maintains its moisture because of the soft gel the psyllium fibre forms.

As a result, the waste remains moist and soft and therefore easier to pass. A soft stool means less chance of diverticular disease and haemorrhoids.

In the case of diarrhoea, because of the soft bulk it forms, psyllium husk helps to provide bulk to the waste matter and slows it down. Most fibre, because it is usually too abrasive, cannot achieve this.

Once things slow down sufficiently the all-important healthy bacteria will start to proliferate again. This is often the catalyst that overcomes diarrhoea which has been caused by a toxic colon. Recent studies have confirmed this.

'Psyllium husks should be the starting point for all symptoms of irritable bowel syndrome.'

This was the recommendation by doctors in Holland who looked into the benefits of increasing fibre in cases of IBS in a recent randomised placebo controlled trial.

It is something I have been advocating for more than 15 years and it is nice to see it being proven in a growing number of studies.

The Dutch study compared the use of psyllium husks against bran fibre in cases of irritable bowel syndrome. They found that psyllium husks had significant benefits for sufferers whereas bran fibre, in most cases, made things worse.

My experience over the last 15 years

This is why I have always recommended psyllium fibre for all sufferers of IBS and constipation because is helps both 'stubborn' and 'sensitive' forms.

It is this unique feature which makes psyllium the best fibre in the world.

It acts like a very gentle broom as it travels through the digestive tract.

The moist environment psyllium creates is also an ideal platform for healthy bacteria to develop.

In the case of diarrhoea, or sensitive irritable bowel, psyllium helps to bind waste matter together and reduce transit time. This gives any good bacteria in the colon a chance to re-establish itself. (If waste matter is moving through too fast, then the good bacteria is often flushed straight through with little chance to survive).

Many, if not most, cases of IBS appear to be linked to some disruption of healthy bacteria in the large colon and finding ways to reverse this situation is the key to relieving symptoms.

It has always been my opinion, and often my experience, that psyllium husks provide this stability that the probiotics need to 'regroup.'

This recent Dutch study would appear to endorse this. To quote the main researcher Dr Niek de Wit: 'It is unlikely that people with IBS would get enough soluble fibre from fruit and other foods to help them. I think adding psyllium to the diet is the best treatment option to start with. In the study, people did this by adding it to things such as yoghurt and it had a real effect.'

Bijkerk CJ et al, Soluble or insoluble fibre in irritable bowel syndrome in primary care? Randomised placebo controlled trial. BMJ 2009;339 (Aug 27)

The synergy of psyllium and probiotics is further enhanced in a recent Japanese trial

In this study, researchers from the Nippon Medical School in Tokyo reported that when sufferers of Ulcerative Colitis were supplemented just with probiotics on their own, there was no significant improvement in the quality of life. It was only when the probiotics were taken with psyllium benefits were shown.

'This was a randomised controlled trial carried out at the Nippon Medical School in Tokyo on the efficacy of symbiotic versus probiotic or prebiotic treatment to improve the quality of life in patients with ulcerative colitis.'

Authors: S. Fujimori, K. Gudis, K. Mitsui, T. Seo, M. Yonezawa, S. Tanaka, A. Tatsuguchi, C. Sakamoto. Doi:10.1016/j.nut.2008.11.017

Friendly bacteria love the moist environment that the psyllium creates. It literally thrives on it. Taking psyllium and probiotics together form a good partnership. This recent research has proven the synergy between these two ingredients which make them an extremely powerful double-act for cleansing your bowels.

But, there is also another type of fibre that operates in a different way to psyllium which can also really help you in your battle to rid yourself of constipation. The name of this fibre is inulin – a truly remarkable ingredient that has so many nutritional benefits.

Recommendation 4:

Inulin – a unique fibre which works to prevent putrefaction in the large colon

Therefore the fourth ingredient is another fibre. The one I recommend is inulin which is commonly found in root vegetables like onions, leeks, chicory, artichokes and agave.

This fibre is different to psyllium in that it doesn't expand and have the 'chamois leather' effect of psyllium. It actually cleanses in a different way which is why the two fibres are so complementary when taken together.

This is how it works. As the food containing the inulin is digested, the inulin passes through the small intestine without getting broken down. Once it arrives at the colon or large intestine, it ferments in a friendly way and is converted into bifidum bacteria, one of the most important strains of friendly bacteria.

This is absolutely brilliant because it is in the large intestine in particular where you need loads of good bacteria. Incidentally, the inulin also acts as a fermentable source of food for other friendly bacteria already present in the colon, so it has a double whammy effect.

Added to that, because it is not converted until it actually reaches the colon, inulin can be a much more stable way of promoting your friendly bacteria than normal probiotics.

This means that inulin is not a probiotic but it is converted to one type of probiotic strain once it arrives in the large colon. This is why it was given the term as being a 'prebiotic' by Professor Glen Gibson from Reading University who was a pioneer of much of the early research on inulin.

Since then there have been numerous studies on inulin which is now known to have a number of other benefits as well as its prebiotic properties.

Throughout this book, I am encouraging you to eat more and more vegetables so that they become not just an addition to your diet but a large percentage of it. Simply just by doing this you will increase your levels of inulin.

However, the actual levels of inulin present in most vegetables these days are quite small, so you have to literally eat loads to get a significant prebiotic, cleansing effect.

Our ancestors and prebiotics

Our plain-dwelling ancestors were big-time eaters of inulin containing plants and prebiotic consumption was significantly higher than today. The type of subsurface plants and bulbs they used to eat in large quantities were onions and agave. Studies have shown that inulin-rich plants dominated the dietary intake of our ancestors with about 60% of their calorific intake coming from such sources.

This would equal a dietary fibre intake of between 250-400gms (their bowels movements must have been prolific) and inulin between 50 and 100gms. Today's recommendation is that we should consume between 8 and 10gms of inulin but to get to even these seemingly low levels would probably require a mountain of vegetables!!

The good news is that these days inulin is available in powder form. It is a white powder and in most cases extracted from chicory. When added to liquid it dissolves almost completely, so you can hardly see it. This makes it easier to take than psyllium but, as I mentioned earlier, it doesn't form the cleansing type of gel that psyllium does. It works in a different way.

By increasing the levels of bifidum bacteria in the colon, inulin can be a great way of reducing the effects of any 'putrefaction' going on and enhance the effects of existing bacteria. I have worked with this wonderful ingredient for more than 15 years and found it absolutely brilliant for keeping my own bowels healthy too!

Taking quite a lot of inulin on its own can make you quite windy at first but usually this settles down after a few days. However, I have always felt that inulin and psyllium work better when taken together. The presence of psyllium clearly has the potential to enhance the prebiotic effect of inulin and, another recent study has shown how these two ingredients actually enhance each other's activities and can be considered to be 'synergistic.' It is my advice therefore that these two ingredients should be taken together with the probiotics.

I now want to move on to the fifth and final ingredient, Magnesium, which is not a fibre or probiotic but a simple – and extremely important – mineral.

Recommendation 5:

Magnesium – a simple mineral - which can be the key to helping you overcome your constipation.

If you are one of those who have been unable to find relief from long term constipation no matter what you try, then this simple mineral could make the difference.

I suspect that if you have been to see your doctor about constipation, then you will have been prescribed some sort of laxative which helps to 'kick start' the peristalsis action. This is fine in the short term, but if you continue down this road, then, as we now know, your bowels will simply get used to the laxative and eventually you will find yourself back to square one – and possibly worse.

However, if you are looking for something to give your new diet a 'helping hand' then a balanced magnesium supplement might be the answer – rather than resorting to laxatives.

Supplementing your new diet with a well balanced magnesium supplement can get you going, comfortably and naturally.

I find that it works best alongside the soluble fibre, psyllium husks. This is because both ingredients work in different ways to improve digestive transit time comfortably and naturally.

Magnesium influences bowel function and some cases of constipation might in fact be a sign that your body is deficient of this crucial mineral.

How Magnesium works

Magnesium encourages water to be drawn into the colon, where it softens stools in the large colon making for a smooth, natural passage. Magnesium is also responsible for the normal functioning of the muscles and this encourages the peristalsis movement.

Magnesium is a mineral – an essential nutrient necessary for a wide range of bodily functions. But studies have shown that even if you are eating normally, you are on the whole likely to be deficient in this vital mineral because you are not getting anywhere near the RDA (recommended daily allowance) from your diet. There is no doubt that many cases of constipation may be due to a deficiency of this important mineral.

By correcting your biochemistry and maintaining adequate levels of magnesium in your body, your bowel movements will become much easier. You'll be able to have an effortless bowel movement at least once a day.

Why is Magnesium deficiency so widespread?

The answer is that the food that you eat today just isn't what it used to be. It is nutritionally weaker and lacks many essential vitamins and minerals. That's because modern farming methods have worn away our top soils by planting the same crop year after year and by growing foods with artificial chemicals, pesticides and herbicides. So the agricultural products are not as rich in nutrients (vitamins, minerals and amino acids) as they should be.

Commercial food processing destroys even more of your food's nutrients. And on top of this, the stress we all face in our day to day lives means that our use of magnesium is accelerated and this can result in 'burn out'. A stressed-out person requires greater requirements of nutrients than a person who is not under a lot of stress.

Magnesium is particularly vulnerable to stress

By correcting your biochemistry and maintaining adequate levels of magnesium in your body, your bowel movements will become much easier.

Well, the good news is that if you are increasing your intake of fresh fruit and vegetables and the majority of this is organic, then you will be vastly increasing your chances of increasing your magnesium levels.

However, in the early stages of changing your diet, if you are finding that things are not moving quite as fast as you feel they should, then taking a magnesium supplement for a while could bring about results.

Taking Magnesium is not like taking a laxative

A laxative is something that would not normally be ingested by the body through your normal diet. It works by 'kick starting' the peristalsis action of the bowels, acting as a purgative. This type of laxative is commonly known to weaken your bowel wall and become habit forming.

On the other hand, magnesium is a natural substance normally supplied in your diet. It works by correcting one of the underlying causes of constipation. When you add magnesium to your daily supplement program (in the dosage you require to get your bowels moving) you are correcting the problem on a nutritional level, preventing constipation from happening.

If you do consider taking a magnesium supplement for a while, then you will probably need to take around 600mg of pure, elemental magnesium each day for a few days to get an effect. You can then taper things down as your diet improves. Taking a supplement which contains a blend of different magnesium salts is probably the best option

So, there you have it. Five different ingredients which you can dip into if you feel you need some help to get things moving. Of course, I am hoping that your new diet will achieve results fast but sometimes, with the busy lives we lead it's not always possible to eat just right. These natural ingredients – taken individually or together - can help bridge any gaps.

But overcoming constipation and clearing your tubes of debris is not all about food – there are some other things you can do to help yourself as well.

CHAPTER 12

Some non-food tips you can do for yourself

If you are serious about your life-changing diet, there are one or two bits of equipment that might make life a bit easier. None of these are essentials but are worth considering.

Bounce your way to better functioning bowels – get a bouncer

There have been a number of studies that have shown that athletes are less prone to constipation than non-athletes. Presumably all the extra 'jarring' spurs the bowels into action and 'kick starts' the peristalsis action.

One way to get that 'jarring' effect without having to pound the streets is to buy a small rebounder (trampoline) which can be folded away into a small cupboard when not in use.

The 'bounce' effect you get from them is not only good for your bowels - it is also good to keep the lymphatic system moving.

As I mentioned earlier in the book, the lymphatic system is an integral and important part of your elimination system. Unlike the heart and blood circulation, the lymphatic system does not have a 'pump' to keep things moving.

Exercise and general activity will encourage the lymph to flow making it more effective as a waste disposer. There have been a number of studies in the last decade which have shown that those people who exercise (moderately) on a regular basis are far less likely to suffer from bowel disease.

Clearly exercise has a beneficial effect on total elimination because it can also help two other parts of the elimination factory – the skin and the lungs. Both work better with exercise. The skin through sweating and the lungs through exhalation.

More exercise means more water! As water is going to be a very important weapon in you fight against unwanted waste in your body, then a really good filter will be well worth the investment.

Purify your system - invest in a water filter

A good filter will remove harmful 'extras' such as fluoride (in some areas) and lead. The best filters are reverse osmosis and are those that fit under the sink and filter your tap water. They cost from around £500.00 to £1000.00 (to include fitting) and around £250.00 pounds per year to service. That's expensive but I believe they are worth it when you consider all the time, effort and money you can spend carting heavy bottles of water from the supermarket.

Also, some of these bottled waters are not quite as pure as we would like them to be! The filter system I use is from The H20 Company. Most suppliers of home filter systems would allow you to pay monthly for a purchase.

Also, proper filtered water gives an added 'freshness' to any drink, both hot and cold. Your daily cuppa never tasted so good!

Feel the cleansing power of organic fruit and vegetables - invest in a juicer

Whilst on the subject of liquids, remember the cleansing, invigorating power of pure organic fruit juices.

In the book I have made reference to the cleansing power of freshly prepared fruit and vegetable juices. Once again, a good juicer does not come cheap. I have purchased a Champion which cost around £250.00. However, I use it daily and so it is money well spent.

These juicers are robust and should last many years. If you do buy one then I also recommend getting an apple slicer and de-corer. It slices and 'de-cores' apples and prepares them for the juicer in one go, which can save you a lot of time. You can get these from IKEA for less than £5.

Keep your skin beautiful and clear – adopt a regular skin brushing programme

This is another activity you can indulge in that can help in the overall cleansing of your system. The main idea of skin brushing is to stimulate the lymphatic system – to help keep it moving and prevent it from stagnating.

You can purchase a suitable brush (with handle) from most pharmacies or stores like The Body Shop.

Skin-brushing is highly effective for preventing the pores getting choked with millions of dead cells. It helps prevent impurities from remaining in the body and relieving the kidneys and liver of some of the work they have to do.

Skin brushing itself – dry of course, not in the bath – will change the health of your whole body. Circulation, skin softness and quality, skin infections and irritations, are all areas of improvement you can look forward to when you make it a regular habit. Regular brushing also means less use of soaps – some of which can be clogging.

The correct technique is to brush in circular strokes all over the body. You start with the soles of your feet; work-up each leg, brushing upwards towards your heart. After the legs you brush the arms, again brushing towards your heart. Then from the top of the shoulders brush downwards and then, finally, brush under your navel upwards – once again towards your heart.

If you do this thoroughly it will take around 10 minutes. Two to three times per week would be good – daily even better. Then, if you are really lucky, your partner will give your back a nice brushing!

Get organised – invest in some food containers for when you are not at home

Being organised is the key. Having a good, air-tight food container will enable you to prepare food at home and take it with you to work or when you are travelling.

Having opted for a delivery of two large boxes of organic vegetables and fruit weekly, I have plenty of options to increase my fruit and veg. However, I have now had to invent creative ways of making sure I use them up efficiently. Taking lots of fruit to work is not a problem but eating vegetables throughout the day – particularly if you're at work is not so easy.

I now take bubble and squeak into work along with my Hippocrates soup so I do find food containers useful. Bubble and squeak helps me keep up my cleansing diet. Try it with hummus, it tastes great. It also stops me relying on baguettes from the bakery round the corner which tended to leave me with that 'bloated' feeling later in the afternoon.

Take one small step…..

I mentioned in Chapter 2 about investing in a small step (or pile of thick books) to have with you in the bathroom to use when going to the loo. The height must be sufficient to raise your knees to a slightly higher level than your hips as this will help to achieve a more complete evacuation. It's worthwhile trying this – but don't give up straight away if it feels a bit strange. You might find it takes a few weeks of perseverance before you get used to it and feel the benefit.

Give your bowels a treat – with a regular massage!

It may sound a bit daft on first hearing, but I recommend anyone to consider this. It will not only help alleviate constipation but – if you do it right and on a regular basis – it can give you more energy as well.

Massaging is a great way to tone and strengthen the muscles in your colon and this can aid in the loosening and removal of stagnant chime that can be causing constipation.

You can massage your colon as you lie on your bed using oils or whilst standing in the shower.

Lying down would of course be the most comfortable. There are now blended aromatherapy oils available which are specifically formulated for colon massage.

To massage – start on the right side down near your appendix. It can be located two inches in from the top of the RIGHT hip and two inches downwards.

Start with small circular or short movements and move upward toward your rib cage. This is the direction your fecal matter travels in your colon.

You can apply pressure using your fingers or knuckles. You may want to start gently and increase your pressure in subsequent days.

When you start your circular massage near your appendix, you are also strengthening your ileocecal valve. (What's that?)

The ileocecal valve is located between the ileum (the last portion of your small intestine) and the cecum (first portion of your large intestine). Its function is to allow digested food materials to pass from the small intestine into your large intestine.

This valve also blocks these waste materials from backing up into your small intestine. It is intended to be a one-way valve, only opening up to allow processed foods to pass through.

If the ileocecal valve is not functioning efficiently then this could affect the even flow of waste matter into the large colon and this in turn could end up being one of the contributors to constipation.

The ileocecal valve will benefit from regular massage.

Massage in the same way (with small, circular motions). Regular massage will help strengthen the ileocecal valve and this will aid in the fight against constipation.

Keep massaging in an upward direction. Once you have reached the rib cage, continue to massage from right to left until you reach the outer point of the left rib cage.

Now continue massaging in a downwards motion two inches in from your LEFT hip towards your groin.

See if you can find five minutes to do this on a daily basis. You will find your constipation easing and an improvement in your overall well being.

As you massage your colon area, take notice if you find areas that have a slight pain or a lot of pain. With areas that have a slight pain, you can work these and probably reduce the pain with daily massages.

With areas of deep pain it might be wise to not continue the massage and consider consulting your GP if the pain persists.

Remember to move your hands in one direction in short strokes upwards then to the left, and then downwards.

A daily colon massage will stimulate both your appendix and your ileocecal valve.

These massages will help to loosen and move faecal matter that is stagnant in your colon. They can be one of those little 'extras' you can do for your bowels that can make all the difference.

CHAPTER 13

Let food be your medicine

Those practitioners like Robert Gray state that all foods apart from vegetables, fruit and honey are mucus forming to some extent. Some mucus foods are to be considered worse than others as I have already stated.

I mentioned in Chapter 6 about Dr. Arnold Ehret and his book The Mucusless Diet and Healing System and how he theorized that all disease is caused by a clogging of the tube and membrane structures within the body due to a build-up of restrictive mucus.

This theory, it would seem, is very similar to the Gerson Therapy which uses copious levels of organic fruit and vegetables to flush and cleanse the body from many diseases including many forms of cancer.

As our understanding of what we put in our mouths grows, our health over time should improve. As Hippocrates said over 2500 years ago, *"Let food be your medicine".*

There is always going to be controversy about what is and isn't healthy food as there are so many vested interests involved - the jury is still out on so many things.

However, there is no controversy about the topic of eating fresh fruit, vegetables and salad type foods. Everyone accepts that good levels are protective against disease.

Scientists are still learning about how different plant oxidants work in the body and I am sure that research is going to increase in this area over the next 20 years. However, different fruit and veg have different attributes and therefore offer different benefits.

This is why eating a variety of fruit and veg is important. Going for all colours of the rainbow appears to be a good recommendation. Following this advice will give your body a broader based support for your overall health and it will also give your digestive system the 'cleansing' effect you are seeking.

So, you could theorise that those foods which tend to be mucus forming are also those that are the precursors to disease if taken as the major part of your diet.

You could then take this a stage further and consider that this is the reason that a growing number of naturopaths and nutritionists believe that many diseases, no matter where they start in the body, are the result of a toxic colon that is gummed up with rotting waste matter which eventually finds its way back into the body as a poison.

Certainly it seems to make sense to suggest that by keeping your bowels working well and clear of obstruction, you can reduce the chance of disease appearing elsewhere in the body. Surely there has to be a certain logic about this statement?

But, in reality, it would be nonsense to recommend that anyone goes on a totally mucus-free diet because this would mean excluding some otherwise healthy foods. The obvious ones I keep mentioning are porridge, eggs and fish.

The secret overall is to focus on those foods where the benefits outweigh the negatives. Oats for example contain gluten and have the potential to be mucus forming but the benefit of their soluble fibre content will generally outweigh the negatives of the mucus effect.

If you are taking oats just for the fibre, then look to alternatives to add to your diet such as linseed or psyllium.

So the secret in keeping a toxic colon at bay is getting the overall balance right and ensuring that the major part of your diet is 'cleansing' rather than mucus forming. This is all you need to do – and it's not difficult. .

Whilst writing this book, I have started to make an effort to become wheat and dairy free. In reality, I ate very little of these two food categories and I have found it very easy to remove them almost totally from my diet. I confess that I find it hard to turn down a tea with milk that someone has made for me but gradually green tea is taking over as my favourite daily tipple. I've realised now how many alternatives there are out there, you just have to look for them and you'll be spoilt for choice.

On the question of soya products, this is the subject of big debate at the moment. The general theory is that if you are going to replace milk, don't rely totally on soya milk as an alternative unless you are being recommended it by a practitioner for specific health reasons. Consider rice and oat milk as well.

If you are not a vegetarian, then the largest proportion of your evening meal should be made up of fresh vegetables and only a small percentage taken up by fish or meat and no red meat if possible.

The diet of our ancestors

In fact the diet of our pre-historic ancestors as I pointed out in Chapter 10, was one of mainly fruits, berries and root vegetables. The image we have of them being largely meat eaters is inaccurate. In fact their diet was pretty cleansing and high in inulin.

Recently there was a food programme on T.V. where a group of middle aged people with the normal middle aged problems of high cholesterol, type 2 diabetes, atherosclerosis, and asthma were taken off somewhere in the wilderness and only allowed to eat fruit, berries and raw vegetables. Even fish was off the menu.

As you can guess, at the end of three weeks, the health outlook for all these people changed. Bowel transit had improved, blood sugars were normal; body fat was down as was cholesterol. As you might expect they were desperate for some 'normal' food but this exercise showed just what could be achieved in extreme circumstances. It really demonstrates 'you are what you eat' and that food can be your medicine.

Okay, it doesn't have to be like that and you cannot be expected to go to such extremes, but it demonstrates the direct and immediate impact diet can have on your body. Too many people today do not consider food to be a medicine. What you put into your mouth and how your digestive system deals with it clearly influences your health.

It is no coincidence that a western diet is linked to higher levels of constipation and colon cancer

Does your existing diet increase your chance of colon cancer?

A recent study has confirmed earlier findings that the high calorie, high mucus forming, low fibre foods associated with the normal Western diet are associated with an increased risk of bowel cancer. This is according to the British charity Cancer Research UK.

"Countries that have had a rapid 'westernisation' of diet, such as Japan, have seen a rapid increase in the incidence of colorectal cancer. Consumption of meat and dairy products in Japan increased ten-fold between the 1950s and 1990s."

The new research, published in the American Journal of Epidemiology, was based on the French cohort of the European Prospective Investigation into Cancer and Nutrition (EPIC) study.

(To explain this: Throughout Europe, there are long term studies underway to determine the effects that different diets have on peoples' health. I believe I am correct in saying that this massive project is being managed from the UK. Different studies, taking place over many years, are being carried out across many countries in Europe. This particular study was carried out in France and relates to diets and their influence on bowel health).

Four dietary patterns were identified by the author of the study.

1. A diet rich in fruit and vegetables, lots of olive oil, and fish. This is fairly similar to a 'Mediterranean diet' and is a living example of a diet which is far less mucus forming than the average UK diet. This is the diet which is considered to be the healthiest for the bowels. In fact the consumption of fish has been shown to have particular benefits and fish oil capsules with high levels of EPA have been shown to be particularly protective.

Also, if you are vegetarian, you are far less likely to get bowel cancer than red meat eaters.

2. A Western diet. This is a diet rich in processed meat, eggs, butter, potatoes, processed grain products, and cheese. This diet was associated with a 39 % increase in bowel disease. Here the percentage of mucus foods is very high.

3. The 'drinker' diet. Here there is an emphasis on alcoholic consumption, snacks, sandwiches and processed meat and pastries. This diet was associated with a 42% increase in bowel disease. As soon as you start to mention pastry type products with high levels of wheat and snacks, you know that the pendulum is swinging rapidly in the wrong direction.

4. 'Meat eaters"   Here the risk rose to 58%. Here the emphasis was on red meat which is notoriously difficult to digest and therefore potentially very mucus forming. I was surprised that the 'meat eaters diet' came out higher than the 'drinkers diet.'

Clearly red meat is one of the major culprits for colon disease and should be reduced right down or even completely removed if you are constipated. You only have to see for yourself how difficult it can be to chew a steak to understand how hard your digestive system has to work to break it down.

As we have seen before, if there is insufficient acid in the stomach to break down the meat sufficiently, problems can then accelerate.

The Mediterranean diet is a living diet that is naturally less mucus forming than the average UK diet and it is one which many of us can now associate with. So, it isn't that difficult to change things around if you really want to.

Although people in Greece and Italy will eat meat and other mucus forming foods, their overall balance is far better than ours.

It is no coincidence that a Mediterranean diet is not only better for our digestive health but also heart health as well. Yet another direct demonstration of how food can have a direct beneficial effect on different parts of your body.

One of the keys to good health is keeping your many miles of tubes and arteries around your body open and clear. This is why I believe the diet I am recommending to you is so good, because it is aimed at doing just that.

CHAPTER 14
What's the hurry?

I want to leave you with one passing thought.

Throughout this book I have talked about getting the balance right in your diet to keep yourself healthy and overcome the constipation that you have been living with.

I have made recommendations throughout this book to take 'time out' when you are eating and to slow things down.

Dr Nick Baylis, therapist and author of the Rough Guide to Happiness argues that there is no activity that isn't improved by slowing it down to at least half or even a quarter of our regular pace. He believes that exercising, eating, speaking, sex; they are dramatically improved by taking our own sweet time.

Eating is no exception.

I really do mean eating when you are quiet and relaxed and not whilst watching the television or even reading the newspaper. By concentrating on what you eat, you can appreciate the texture and the taste better and, just as important, you can make sure it is probably 'liquidised' before swallowing.

Life is just too busy these days with everyone rushing around, it is no wonder most people middle aged and above have some type of digestive disorder. Eating when stressed is a recipe for disaster for your digestive system in the long term.

Many of us now eat on the move without giving our digestive systems a chance to do their jobs properly.

When I was young you often heard people telling you not to rush your food. My paternal grandfather lived until he was 96. I shared a house with him in my early teenage years and I learned so much from him. One of the statements he was famous for after we had eaten was 'let your food go down.' He was often chastising me for trying to rush from the table to go and play with my friends. He was a hard working man, and no-one had ever advised him how to look after himself but like a lot of people born in Victorian times, he seemed to know what was right for his body intuitively. He was, perhaps, more in tune with his body than we are today. Certainly after every meal, no matter how small, he would sit quietly, either at the table or in his easy chair, and not move for around ten minutes. He was convinced that you needed to give your digestive system some quiet time to process the food that had just been presented to it.

It is perhaps not surprising therefore to learn that he also chewed his food incredibly slowly – in fact painfully slowly for a child who had to wait until he had finished eating before being allowed to get down from the table.

So, what has this to do with constipation? Well, perhaps quite a lot. If your food is not broken down properly during the early part of the digestive process, then your whole digestive system, including the functioning of your bowels, will be under stress and will not work according to plan.

As I have tried to emphasise time and time again in this book, your eating processes should not be rushed.

Try to put time aside at meal times so that you can think about the food you are eating. Try and enjoy the process without looking at it as purely a functional role that you need to get through as quickly as possible.

Easier said than done, I know, but it's worth working on.

So I hope this book has been interesting for you and more importantly, useful. What started out as one of my small reports on bowel health turned out to be something a little longer and more detailed! Proof in itself that you cannot dismiss regular, long term constipation as an isolated problem confined to your colon.

As with all health issues, there is the argument about treating the symptoms or the causes.

As I have a company that specialises in natural products it is not surprising that I favour treating the causes with food and/or natural nutrients whenever possible.

Understanding those nutrients and foods that can keep you healthy can give you immense power over your own destiny rather than leaving others to do it for you. In fact, as many of you have found, doctors are just too busy to look at your health as a whole. It is their focus to look just at those symptoms that are placed before them and opt for the quick fix.

Of course, prevention is by far the best approach to health in general. It is your job to try to look after your overall health and prevent disease from taking place in the first place. This means preventing constipation if you can and looking after your digestive system.

For those of you who are already severely constipated I hope that this book will point you in a new direction which will not only give you long-term relief but also the knowledge to take control over your own bowel health - because this could be the key to your overall well-being.

Further reading:

Good Gut Healing by Kathryn Marsden. As it says on the cover – it's a no-nonsense guide to bowel and digestive disorders.

The Gerson Therapy What I like about this book and the Gerson therapy is that it demonstrates the power of food and how it can cleanse and heal your body.

A Time to Heal by Beata Bishop. This is one person's experience of healing her body through the Gerson Therapy.

Lose Wheat Lose Weight by Antoinette Savill. If you want to know more about how you can 'bung up' your system with too much wheat – this book is worth a read.